WINNICOTT

Winnicott

Adam Phillips

Harvard University Press
Cambridge, Massachusetts

Library of Congress Cataloging-in-Publication Data

Phillips, Adam.
  Winnicott.

  Bibliography: p.
  1. Child analysis.   2. Winnicott, D. W. (Donald
Woods), 1896–1971.   I. Title.   II. Series
RJ504.2.P48 1989   155.4   88-28390
ISBN 0-674-95360-6 (cloth)
ISBN 0-674-95361-4 (paper)

For PAUL VAN HEESWYK

CONTENTS

ACKNOWLEDGEMENTS

This book is the result of several years' learning and teaching psychoanalysis, in which innumerable debts have been incurred. I owe a great deal, in particular to Masud Khan and Christopher Bollas from whom I learnt versions of psychoanalysis that were inspiring and intelligible.

The prompt criticism and enthusiastic interest of Geoffrey Summerfield and Hugh Haughton made the writing of this book possible, as did the assistance of Eileen Joyce. The book has benefited from a variety of suggestions from Alex Coren, Morian Roberts, Charles Rycroft, Michel Gribinski, Richard Poirier, Michael Neve, Jimmy Britton, Geoffrey Weaver and George Moran. I would also like to thank Madeleine Davis and the Winnicott Publications Committee for their support of the project, and the librarians of the New York Hospital-Cornell Medical Center for their help. The editors of *Raritan* and the *Nouvelle Revue de Psychoanalyse* have given invaluable support to my work.

My own sense of what psychoanalysis is about evolved in conversation with the person to whom this book is dedicated.

London, June 1988

'The first lesson that innocent Childhood affords me is – that it is an instinct of my Nature to pass out of myself, and to exist in the form of others.

'The second is – not to suffer any one form to pass into ME and become a usurping Self in the disguise of what the German Pathologists call a FIXED IDEA.'

S. T. Coleridge

'I have followed my inclination rather than consulted my ability.'

Ralph Waldo Emerson

Introduction

'Health is much more difficult to deal with
than disease.'

D. W. Winnicott

In a talk given in 1945 to the sixth form of St Paul's School,
Donald Winnicott described his experience, as a schoolboy,
of discovering Darwin's *Origin of Species*:

> I could not leave off reading it. At the time I did not
> know why it was so important to me, but I see now
> that the main thing was that it showed that living
> things could be examined scientifically with the corol-
> lary that gaps in knowledge and understanding need not
> scare me. For me this idea meant a great lessening of
> tension and consequently a release of energy for work
> and play.[1]

Darwin had examined living things to explain their relation
to each other. He realized that gaps in the evolutionary
record were merely interruptions in the historical evidence
for the continuity of species. Just as Freud would later
describe the repressed histories of the individuals he treated,
Darwin had reconstructed the invisible histories of species.
Gaps in the evidence were openings, and both Darwin and
Freud had been able to tell persuasive, apparently coherent
stories about them. Winnicott implies by his remarks that
he needed to be able not to close the gaps, but to find a way
of examining them. They could be potential spaces for the
imagination. He was to be preoccupied, as we shall see, by

1

the idea of gaps, those 'spaces between' where there was room for the play of speculation.

In the master-plot of human development that he worked on for over forty years, Winnicott tried to explain how the individual grows, through dependence, towards a personal way of being, how he becomes at once ordinary and distinctive according to the sense he has of himself, and how the early environment makes this possible. Growth was this ongoing task of psychosomatic integration. He was to stress the need for continuity of care – 'good-enough mothering' – to sustain what he called the 'going on being', the 'life-line' of the infant, at the earliest stages of its life. He would talk, enigmatically for a psychoanalyst, of instinctual life as a possible 'complication' in the individual's more fundamental needs for relationship. He would regard illness as the inhibition of that potential spontaneity that for him characterized the aliveness of a person. And he would come to think of psychopathology as originating from the breaks in continuity, the distractions in a person's early development: gaps caused by the intrusions and deprivations and natural catastrophes of childhood, most of which he saw as resulting from failures of parental provision. There were things the child had experienced but could not make satisfying sense of, and so find a place for in himself. For the infant who waits too long for his mother, for example, 'the only real thing is the gap; that is to say, the death or the absence, or the amnesia.'[2]

In Winnicott's view experience was traumatic for the child if it was incomprehensible, beyond the child's grasp. The onus was on the mother, at first, to present the world to the infant in manageable doses. And the onus on those helping mothers and infants, Winnicott believed, was to protect this process. 'If it be true, or even possible,' he writes, 'that the mental health of every individual is founded by the mother in her living experience with her infant, doctors and nurses can make it their first duty not to interfere. Instead of trying to teach mothers how to do what in fact cannot be taught, paediatricians must come sooner or later to recognize a good mother when they see one and then make sure that she gets full opportunity to grow to her job.'[3]

Winnicott's work was devoted to the recognition and description of the good mother, and the use of the mother–infant relationship as the model of psychoanalytic treatment. And he often took for granted that what mothers did naturally, 'what in fact cannot be taught', was a model for the skill of the psychoanalyst.

He examined, in particular, the paradox of traumatic experiences that were formative by virtue of their eluding the self, and the mother's role in facilitating in her infant a self available for personal experience. But Winnicott was to use the concept of the Self in an idiosyncratic and sometimes mystifying way that was not obviously compatible with traditional psychoanalytic theory. 'A word like "self"', he writes, 'naturally knows more than we do; it uses us and can command us.'[4] We will gather from the contexts in which he was used by this powerful word that he was asserting the presence of something essential about a person that was bound up with bodily aliveness, yet remained inarticulate and ultimately unknowable: perhaps like an embodied soul. 'At the centre of each person', Winnicott writes, 'is an incommunicado element, and this is sacred and most worthy of preservation.'[5] This Self that he will describe as 'permanently non-communicating' fits uneasily, of course, with the notion of psychoanalysis as primarily an interpretative practice.

The individual's Self was endangered, above all, Winnicott believed, by precocious adaptation to the environment. In *The Origin of Species* Darwin had noted what he called the 'intermediate' or 'transitional gradations' in the development of species, and the role of the environment in this process. He had realized the value, for survival, of individual diversity and variation, but also the need for the organism to comply with the demands of its environment. Organisms had to conform and adapt but also individuate prolifically in order to increase their chances of survival. Innovation and adaptation were mutually necessary, as those who were finally unable to adapt to their environment would not survive. In Winnicott's theory of human development it is the mother, as the first environment, who 'actively adapts' to the needs of her infant. In Winnicott's terms the child has a natural right, initially, to use the mother ruthlessly for the recognition and gratification that his development requires. 'Without someone specifically orientated to his needs,' he writes, 'the infant cannot find a working relation to external reality.'[6] In time the mother will gradually limit her availability and so 'disillusion' the child, and the child will become concerned about the consequences of his ruthlessness. But Winnicott, as we shall see, is committed to an idea of 'natural' processes of development – derived from Darwinian biology – that the mother can adapt to and foster by her responsive attention. The word 'natural', as we shall also see, does a lot of devious work in Winnicott's writing. It could betray him sometimes – when he refers, for example, to 'the part the woman plays in nature's comic opera'[7] – into a sentimentality that he was otherwise fiercely suspicious of.

The first relationship, in Winnicott's account, was one of reciprocity rather than overwhelming conflict or submission. But if the mother was unable, for reasons to do with her own development, to adapt to her infant's needs and was, herself, intrusively demanding, she would foster a precocious compliance in the child. To manage the demands of the mother, and to protect the True Self of personal need and preoccupation, the child would construct what Winni-

cott called a False Self. By introducing a language of reciprocity into the story of early human development
Winnicott revised part of Darwin's account. He reverses the
Darwinian equation by suggesting that human development
was an often ruthless struggle against compliance with the
environment. And this struggle was enacted in his writing
where we find innovations in psychoanalytic theory and
technique followed by explicit assertions of the continuity
of his work with a more orthodox psychoanalytic tradition.
We will see, in fact, a certain disingenuousness in the way
Winnicott disguises his radical departures from Freud.
'Mature adults', he wrote, 'bring vitality to that which is
ancient, old and orthodox, by recreating it after destroying
it.'[8] With blithe defiance Winnicott recreated, often beyond
recognition, the work of everyone who influenced him.

Compliance was a crucial issue for Winnicott because of
the fact of dependence. The infant relies on the mother's
firm attentiveness for his survival. And the mother in turn
depends upon the people around her that she needs. There
is, as Winnicott once famously said, no such thing as a
baby: 'If you show me a baby you certainly show me also
someone caring for a baby, or at least a pram with someone's
eyes and ears glued to it. One sees a "nursing couple".'[9]
Winnicott would derive everything in his work, including a
theory of the origins of scientific objectivity and a revision
of psychoanalysis, from this paradigm of the developing
mother–infant relationship. He would elaborate what it was
in the mother that the child depended upon, and this would
lead him to questions that were rarely addressed in psychoanalytic theory: what do we depend on to make us feel
alive, or real? Where does our sense come from, when we
have it, that our lives are worth living? Winnicott
approached these issues through the observation – one of
his favoured words – of mothers and infants, and what
became in time the 'transitional space' between them. And

5

he would be committed to linking these observations with insights derived from psychoanalysis. As the first paediatrician in England to train as a psychoanalyst, he was uniquely placed to compare his observations with the always reconstructed, retrospective histories of psychoanalytic treatment.

What went on between the mother and her infant was to be the source of Winnicott's most striking and characteristic insights. But it would be part of his incompatibility with Freud that these insights – the connection, for example, between infantile ruthlessness and adult sexuality – were rarely linked up by him with the place of the erotic in adult life. Fathers tend to turn up in his writing in brackets or parentheses. His most important theoretical contributions to psychoanalysis – transitional phenomena, primary creativity, ruthlessness, the anti-social tendency, the True and False Self – are never described in terms of the difference between the sexes.

Freud, though, had paid little attention in his work to the nursing couple or the details of infant care. He had invented a setting and treatment that were unwittingly reminiscent of early maternal care and he had also, of course, written of the dependent relationship recreated in psychoanalytic treatment. While he had acknowledged the significance, for later development, of the helplessness of the human infant and its precocious immaturity at birth, he had not given this helplessness the centrality it was later to assume for child analysts and the object-relations theorists who thought of themselves as continuing his work. It was the Oedipus Complex – the three-person relationship – not the infant's early dependent vulnerability, that Freud saw as the crux of psychoanalysis. Though he worked out an essential pre-Oedipal schema of development, he put relatively little emphasis on the first relationship with the mother. And he tended to assume a certain developmental achievement in his patients that Winnicott would have questioned. From his case-histories it seems that Freud believed his patients had more or less successfully negotiated the 'long period' of helplessness and entered into the disappointing rigours of incestuous desire.

Freud was interested in the adult's struggle with incompatible and unacceptable desires which he saw as the transformed derivatives of the child's desire for his parents. This desire, that Freud referred to as infantile sexuality, was the precursor of and paradigm for adult sexuality. Out of a profound ambivalence, in Freud's view, the individual constructed an always precarious sexual identity, whereas for Winnicott, out of an always paradoxical involvement with others, the individual gathers the sense of a self he was born with as a potential. Where Freud was concerned with the individual's compromised possibilities for satisfaction, for Winnicott this is only part of a larger issue of the individual's possibilities for personal authenticity, what he will call 'feeling real'. In Winnicott's writing culture can facilitate growth, like the mother; for Freud it prohibits and frustrates like the father. In Freud's view man is divided and driven, by the contradictions of his desire, into frustrating involvement with others. In Winnicott man can only find himself in relation with others, and in the independence gained through acknowledgement of dependence. For Freud, in short, man was the ambivalent animal; for Winnicott he would be the dependent animal, for whom development – the only 'given' of his existence – was the attempt to become 'isolated without being insulated'. Prior to sexuality as the unacceptable there was helplessness. Dependence was the first thing, before good and evil.

In the *Three Essays on Sexuality* (1905) Freud gives his account of the child's earliest developmental needs, the blueprint for all the competing psychoanalytic stories of human development that were to follow. In the first essay he makes a simple distinction that was to be important in the psychoanalysis of children. 'Let us', he writes, 'call the person from whom sexual attraction proceeds the sexual object and the act towards which the instinct tends the sexual aim.' The first object of desire, Freud goes on to say, is for both sexes the mother. But the object, who is at first the mother, Freud claims is merely 'soldered on' to the instinct. That is to say – and this is more obviously true of adult sexuality – there is for Freud no necessary connection between the instinct and its object, for which substitutes can easily be found. In this view the child's, and later the adult's, primary commitment is to the instinct and its satisfaction, not to a specific relationship. In fact, in Freud's view, the infant turns to the mother almost grudgingly out of the inability to be self-satisfied. In other words, dependence was imagined by Freud as a concession on the part of the infant. He comes, in a state verging on disappointment, to a belated awareness of the mother, who is literally an object to relieve the tension born of desire. The infant is conceived of as originally an omnipotent, exploitative hedonist.[10]

With the advent of child analysis, and in particular with the work of Melanie Klein, the earliest stages of this object-relation with the mother came into focus in psychoanalysis for the first time. Instead of the discrete separation of subject and object, of the infant and its mother, the relational matrix became the object of attention. Different accounts of the child's emotional life began to emerge and more specific questions were asked about the place of the mother in the infant's world. Considering children's play as analogous to the free-associations of adults, Klein applied her version of the classical psychoanalytic technique to the treatment of very young children. She interpreted their play and constructed unprecedented and revealing pictures of what she called the child's internal world. Stressing one aspect in particular of infantile sexuality, the infant's sadism, she was the first to formulate, though often in a dense psychoanalytic language of her own, the passionate intensity of early emotional life. As we shall see, her theories of primitive emotional development, and the significance of the child's destructiveness in the process, were to be crucial for Winnicott. His work, in fact, cannot be understood without reference to Klein. It is a continuous, and sometimes inexplicit, commentary on and critique of her work. The importance of the internal world and its objects, the elaborate and pervasive power of fantasy, the central notion of primitive greed – all these ideas Winnicott takes over from Klein and uses in his own way. As we shall see, they evolved different narratives of the developmental process and the mother's contribution to it. But her stringent theoretical positions, and the collusive devotion of her followers, provoked him without dispelling his own idiosyncratic approach.

Winnicott shared with Klein a fundamental belief in the decisive importance of the earliest stages of development. But from the very beginning, he claimed, the infant sought contact with a person, not simply instinctual gratification from an object. The infant starts life as a profoundly sociable being: he clamours for intimacy, not only for relief of tension – for relatedness, not simply for satisfaction. In fact satisfaction is only possible in a context of relatedness to the mother. 'It is not instinctual satisfaction', he writes, 'that makes a baby begin to be, to feel that life is real, to find life worth living.'[11] It was maternal care, he believed, that made it possible for the infant self to be enriched, as opposed to overwhelmed, by instinctual experience. It was the mother's essential role to protect the self of her infant; instincts served the self, in Winnicott's view, they did not constitute it. It was 'the self that must precede the self's use of instinct; the rider must ride the horse, not be run away with.'[12] It was the 'mother's job' to ensure that this happened.

Freud had said that the rider must guide the horse in the direction in which the horse wants to go. He was prescient in his sense that his insistence on the central and subversive importance of sexuality would threaten everyone's allegiance to psychoanalysis. Initiated by Klein, and reformulated by Winnicott, it was to be part of the contribution of what became known as the British School of object-relations theorists, to translate psychoanalysis from a theory of sexual desire into a theory of emotional nurture. It was as though the adult had been usurped by the infant. With the arrival of Melanie Klein in England in 1926, with the work of John Bowlby and Winnicott himself with children evacuated during the war, and with the insights derived from Anna Freud's version of child analysis, a new picture emerged in psychoanalysis of the significance of early relationships for the individual's development. Just as women were being encouraged to stay at home again after their crucial work during the war, coercive and convincing theories about the importance for children of continuous mothering, of the potential dangers of separation, began to be published which could easily be used to persuade them to stay there.[13] In British psychoanalysis after the war there was not so much a return to Freud, as there had been in France with the work of Lacan, as a return to Mother.

II

Under the aegis, though not the leadership, of Winnicott, a Middle Group emerged within the British Psychoanalytical Society. Strongly influenced by child analysis, but not exclusively allied with the work of either Klein or Anna Freud, these analysts – of whom Masud Khan, Charles Rycroft, Marion Milner, John Klauber and Peter Lomas are the most distinguished – formed no school or training of their own. Committed to pluralism rather than hero-worship, their work coheres around a more eclectic developmental model. Coming, broadly speaking, from an empirical rather than a dialectical tradition, their work is characterized by an interest in observation and empathy, a suspicion of abstraction and dogmatism, and a belief in people's ability to make themselves known and be understood. Their theoretical papers refer continually to clinical work; there are few dazzling feats of interpretation or knowingness, and concern for the patient is expressed without irony. Imagination was a necessary term in their more or less shared conceptual vocabulary. Although obliquely influenced by Existentialism, the Middle Group tended to draw their redescriptions of Freud from biology, ethology and literature rather than from linguistics and continental philosophy. Darwin, rather than Hegel or Nietzsche, was a presiding spirit in their work. There was no radical intent in their theory-making. In their writings they did not make comprehensive theoretical assertions, nor was the tone one of shrewd enlightened dismay about the human condition.

For Winnicott, and those who were influenced by his work, psychoanalytic treatment was not exclusively interpretative, but first and foremost the provision of a congenial milieu, a 'holding environment' analogous to maternal care. What Paul Ricoeur has called the 'hermeneutic of suspicion' in Freud's work, is replaced by the attempt to establish an analytic setting in which the patient does not undergo authoritative translation – having his unconscious fed back to him, as it were – but is enabled by the analyst, as Winnicott wrote, 'to reveal himself to himself'. To begin with, the analyst is a certain kind of host: psychoanalysis, he wrote, 'is not just a matter of interpreting the repressed unconscious [but] . . . the provision of a professional setting for trust, in which such work may take place'.[14] Interpreta-

11

tion, as part of the setting, aims to recognize and reconstruct what was absent in the parental provision, what early developmental needs were unacknowledged. The risk was that interpretation in analysis would be formative in a way that actually pre-empted the patient's own half-formed thoughts and feelings. Interpretation could be merely a way of hurrying – on the analyst's behalf – and analysis, like development, was, for Winnicott, about people taking their own time.

Cure, Winnicott wrote, 'at its root means care', care in the service of personal development. The therapist must have 'a capacity . . . to contain the conflicts of the patient, that is to say to contain them and to wait for their resolution in the patient instead of anxiously looking round for a cure'.[15] Cure was not something that the therapist did to the patient. In his consultations with children Winnicott found that the significant moment was the one in which the patient surprised himself. In fact the development of a capacity to be surprised by oneself could be said to be one of the aims of Winnicottian analysis. A surprise, of course, eludes the expectations made possible by a body of theory. It is a release from compliance. From his case-histories it is clear that Winnicott as an analyst was able to be convinced by his own surprises as well as the surprises of his patients.[16] Though psychoanalysts have written a lot about pleasure, Winnicott is one of the few that allows himself to be seen, in his writing, getting pleasure from what he does. And this, I think, is of a piece with one of his major contributions, which was to have evolved a genuinely collaborative model of psychoanalytic treatment in which the analyst creates a setting that also makes possible the patient's self-interpretations. Health for Winnicott was to do with the mutuality of relationship:

> A sign of health in the mind is the ability of one
> individual to enter imaginatively and accurately into

the thoughts and feelings and hopes and fears of another person; also to allow the other person to do the same to us . . . When we are face to face with a man, woman or child in our speciality, we are reduced to two human beings of equal status.[17]

Interestingly, Winnicott's definition of health here echoes John Stuart Mill's definition of the imagination as the ability to 'enter the mind and circumstance of another being'. Though obviously prone to sentimental mystification, the idea of the reciprocity of the professional relationship was a new note in psychoanalysis, as were other of Winnicott's controversial and apparently whimsical pronouncements. When he wrote, for example, that 'we are poor indeed if we are only sane';[18] or that 'true neurosis is not necessarily an illness . . . we should think of it as a tribute to the fact that life is difficult';[19] or that 'even when our patients do not get cured they are grateful to us for seeing them as they are',[20] he was, in his own blithe and unbeglamoured way, radically revising conventional psychoanalytic pieties. A certain arch honesty, an often wilfully benign astuteness is part of Winnicott's distinctive style.

Although occasionally coy, his prose has none of the dreary earnestness or mystifying jargon that mars psychoanalytic writing after Freud and Ferenczi. His thought reflects, as André Green has written, 'above all, a richly alive experiencing rather than an erudite schematizing'. Because his papers were presented to a wide range of audiences, and because he was intent on being understood rather than copied, there is little arcane language in his writing. Instead there is a handful of idiosyncratic terms – holding, using, playing, feeling real, illusion and disillusion, true and false self, transitional phenomena – that, as we shall see, make up his developmental theory. What he refers

13

to continually as the developmental process is the idol around which his work is organized. And the prominence of verbal nouns reflects his preoccupation with process rather than conclusion (he was, Masud Khan has written, 'always mobile'). The notorious 'simplicity' of his language, however, is problematic. Though acutely aware himself of the way words are mobile – 'they have etymological roots, they have a history: like human beings they have a struggle sometimes to establish and maintain identity'[21] – he uses certain key terms as though they had no history in psychoanalytic thought. And while he recommends simple interpretations in analysis – 'I never use long sentences unless I am very tired'[22] – his interventions in his case-histories can be elaborate and surprisingly abstract.

The genre of simplicity in which Winnicott writes, a wry version of pastoral, is in fact a kind of elusiveness. But the shrewd ingenuousness of his writing, unprecedented in the psychoanalytic tradition, is consistent with one of his therapeutic aims: to protect the privacy of the self in the making of personal sense and, by the same token, personal non-sense. 'In the relaxation that belongs to trust and to the acceptance of the professional reliability of the therapeutic setting . . . there is room for the idea of unrelated thought sequences which the analyst will do well to accept as such, not assuming the existence of a significant thread.'[23] The need of the self to be both intelligible and hidden that he found in his patients is reflected in his style. There has never been a strong surrealist tradition in England but there has of course been a unique tradition of nonsense. And though Winnicott sounds like no one else writing in the psychoanalytic tradition, he can often sound curiously like Lewis Carroll. It is, in fact, part of his irreverence as a psychoanalyst to be entertaining. Only Winnicott could have written as a footnote to one of his most important papers: 'When the analyst knows that the patient carries a revolver, then, it seems to me, this work cannot be done.'[24]

Though we can hear something of E. M. Forster, or his near contemporary Stevie Smith, in Winnicott's writing, there are no comparable echoes of previous psychoanalytic writers. He struggles to conceal the fact that he often writes uneasily in the psychoanalytic tradition, against the grain of its prevailing forms of seriousness and its fantasies of methodical rigour. His writing has its roots in the English romanticism of Wordsworth, Coleridge and Lamb (and has illuminating parallels, odd though it may seem, with the essays of Emerson and the work of William James). Much of his own work deviates from Freudian metapsychology, and unlike Klein and Anna Freud his work does not derive from specifically identifiable Freudian texts. As previous commentators have remarked: 'Winnicott preserves tradition in a curious fashion, largely by distorting it ... [with] his elusive mode of presentation and his absorption yet transformation of theoretical predecessors.'[25] By recontextualizing crucial terms, he will gloss over their theoretical history. He will describe psychotherapy as a form of playing – 'it has to do with two people playing together'[26] – and at the same time express a marked preference for open-ended games in which play is not circumscribed by agreed-upon rules. In the Squiggle game, his most famous technical innovation, he invites a child to complete a rudimentary doodle that he does on a sheet of blank paper. By responding to the demand and turning the squiggle into something recognizable and shareable, the child offers a sample of his internal world. The repertoire of the child's possible responses is not circumscribed by the therapist. It cannot be calculated. In this reciprocal free-association, this 'game without rules', Winnicott saw the therapeutic potential of a traditional children's game, and adapted it to his psychoanalytic purposes. The charm and immediacy of his use of the technique described in his *Therapeutic Consultations in Child Psychiatry* could be as irresistible to the reader as it was to the child. It was Winnicott's vitality, his flair, that was unprecedented in psychoanalysis, and that created suspicion. By virtue of being new people, infants and young children can be difficult to understand. He could seem to embody a peculiarly modern but misleading ideal of perfect communication with children. There was something 'magical', his critics thought, in the fluency of his contact with the children he saw, as though all one could learn from his clinical accounts was that one was unable to be Winnicott. It will become clear that Winnicott had to be subtly pragmatic in his use of the psychoanalytic tradition. Sometimes he could allow himself to be idiosyncratic only by appearing to comply.

He was, however, explicit about his method of writing papers, which is, in the most interesting way, of a piece with his developmental theory. Introducing a radically innovatory paper to the British Psychoanalytical Society in 1945, he said:

> I shall not first give an historical survey and show the development of my ideas from the theories of others, because my mind does not work that way. What happens is that I gather this and that, here and there, settle down to clinical experience, form my own theories, and then, last of all, interest myself to see where I stole what. Perhaps this is as good a method as any.[27]

In the first sentence he refuses to comply with the way psychoanalytic papers are conventionally organized. He assumes influences are at work – 'I gather this and that, here and there' – and he takes it for granted that in forming his own theories he will discover an indebtedness. He does not, it should be noted, refer to borrowing (on which subject psychoanalysis has always been silent) but to stealing.[28] In his unique theory of delinquency, which he calls the anti-social tendency, Winnicott suggests, as we will see, that the child steals in symbolic form only what once belonged to him by right. The child is unwittingly trying to make up for a deprivation he experienced in the original commonwealth of his relationship with the mother, and he is alerting the environment to this fact. For Winnicott the anti-social act, like a regression in psychoanalytic treatment, is a return to the point at which the environment failed the child. He returns to find where what he hasn't got has come from, to the gaps in himself. Winnicott's method of writing papers, so recognizably close to ordinary experience, enacts this process.

As we trace the development of Winnicott's work we will find his evolving description of the mother–infant relationship mirrored by his own relationship with the psychoanalytic tradition. Like the infant's benign exploitation of the mother, which he describes, he will use the tradition according to his needs in the making of his own personal sense. He will suggest in one of his most remarkable late papers, 'The Use of an Object and Relating through Identification' (1969),[29] that the object only becomes real by being hated; the infant can only find the world around him substantial through his ultimately unsuccessful attempts to destroy it. Winnicott will test the resilience of the body of psychoanalytic knowledge in the development of his most recondite concept, the personal Self. Perhaps in becoming himself the psychoanalytic writer will, of necessity, have a delinquent relationship to the tradition, using it as he needs it. Winnicott, anyway, made it impossible for us to copy him: he is exemplary as a psychoanalyst, by being inimitable.

Metaphor

1 What We Call the Beginning

'. . . there is no absolute tendency to
progression, excepting from favourable
circumstances!'

Charles Darwin

The autobiography that Winnicott started to write in the
last years of his life, entitled 'Not Less Than Everything',
began with a description of his own death. On the inside
cover of the notebook he wrote:

T. S. Eliot   'Costing not less than everything'
T. S. Eliot   'What we call the beginning is often the end
And to make an end is to make a beginning.
The end is where we start from.'

Prayer

D. W. W.   Oh God! May I be alive when I die.[1]

He then begins his autobiography with the sentence, 'I died.'
It is not surprising that Winnicott, as a man in his seventies,
should be preoccupied by his own death. Nor, in a way, that
he should take his grand title from Eliot's description at the
end of the last of his *Four Quartets*, 'Little Gidding', of 'A
condition of complete simplicity/(Costing not less than
everything)'. What is striking, though, is his wish to be alive
– he does not say conscious – at his own death, to be there
to experience, as it were, his own absence. His prayer is a

19

demand, in the form of a question, that what might seem to be a contradiction could be a paradoxical possibility.

In one of the last psychoanalytic papers he wrote, 'Fear of Breakdown'[2] (published in 1973, two years after his death), Winnicott proposed something that 'turns out to be very simple. I contend that clinical fear of breakdown is the fear of a breakdown that has already been experienced.' What happened in the past can only be known about by being projected into the future as a fear. Winnicott links this with the fear of death:

> Little alteration is needed to transfer the general thesis of fear of breakdown to a specific fear of death. This is perhaps a more common fear, and one that is absorbed in the religious teachings about an afterlife, as if to deny the fact of death.
>
> When fear of death is a significant symptom the promise of an afterlife fails to give relief, and the reason is that the patient has a compulsion to look for death. Again, it is the death that happened but was not experienced that is sought.
>
> When Keats was 'half in love with easeful death' he was, according to the idea that I am putting forward here, longing for the ease that would come if he could 'remember' having died; but to remember he must experience death now.[3]

Winnicott characteristically joins up the extreme, fear of breakdown, with the 'more common' fear of death. In his autobiographical account he wanted to be present at his own death. He feared the death he might not experience, the death that might happen without his being alive to it. But the patient who compulsively looks for death is reaching in this way to a memory of a previous death.

The death he describes in 'Fear of Breakdown' as having already happened is the psychic death of the infant, what he

20

calls the 'primitive agony', of an excessive early deprivation that the infant can neither comprehend nor escape from. This intolerable absence of the mother was beyond the infant's capacity to assimilate. It was included as part of the infant's total life experience, but it could not be integrated, it had no place. Beyond a certain point in time the infant, in a sense, was no longer there, he became insentient because he did not have an ego sufficiently developed to encompass, and so account for, the waiting inflicted upon him. He could not hold his belief in his mother's existence alive in his mind:

> The feeling of the mother's existence lasts x minutes. If the mother is away more than x minutes, then the imago fades, and along with this the baby's capacity to use the symbol of the union ceases. The baby is distressed, but this distress is soon mended because the mother returns in x+y minutes. In x+y minutes the baby has not become altered. But in x+y+z minutes the baby has become traumatized. In x+y+z minutes the mother's return does not mend the baby's altered state. Trauma implies that the baby has experienced a break in life's continuity ... Madness here simply means a break-up of whatever may exist at the time of a personal continuity of existence. After 'recovery' from x+y+z deprivation a baby has to start again permanently deprived of the root which could provide continuity with the personal beginning.[4]

A person who had endured this primitive agony might be driven to pursue in the future those significant events – anti-experiences, as it were – which he was unable to include or make sense of in the past. Events without context, they had merely happened. But they had been registered in some way and still had to be located for development to start up again. What was registered, unconsciously in Winnicott's view, was an interruption, a blanking out, an absence in the person's self-experience. Winnicott would write of the Unconscious as, among other things, a place where deprivations were kept.

As development was imperative for the individual, what counted as an experience for Winnicott was anything that contributed to a person's sense of their own growth. 'Each individual', he wrote, 'starts and develops and becomes mature; there is no adult maturity apart from previous development. This development is extremely complex, and it is continuous from birth or earlier right up to and through adulthood and old age.'[5] One of the aims of psychoanalysis was to re-establish continuity with whatever constituted the patient's 'personal beginning'. At the end of his life Winnicott was preoccupied by the final experience he might be unable to have, and by understanding the earliest deprivations that could make people feel that they had not begun to exist. We will see Winnicott thinking along what will become familiar lines of the relationship between the continuous and the interrupted, the present and the absent, the simple and the complicated in a person's life.

For Freud the aim of the organism was to die in its own way. Winnicott, who would evolve a quite different sense of what a life was, would add to this that the individual's aim was to live in his own way, which included for him the ultimate non-compliant act of being alive at his death.

II

Donald Woods Winnicott was born on 7 April 1896 in Plymouth. Named after his mother's father, he was the youngest child and only son of Frederick and Elizabeth Winnicott. The Winnicotts already had two daughters, Cathleen and Violet, who were, respectively, five and six when he was born. Winnicott was to grow up, as he would later write, 'in a sense ... an only child with multiple mothers and with father extremely preoccupied in my younger years with town as well as business matters'. John Frederick Winnicott was forty-one when his son was born, and it is a not uninteresting detail, in the light of his son's future interests, that he was by profession what was then still called a merchant, specializing in women's corsetry. A successful public man, he was twice Mayor of Plymouth (1906–7, 1921–2), a JP, and he was knighted in 1924. Among other public honours in Plymouth he was Chairman of the Chamber of Commerce, Manager of the Plymouth Hospital Committee, and in 1934 was given the freedom of the city. But he was, his son wrote, 'sensitive about his lack of education (he had had learning difficulties) and he always said that because of this he had not aspired to Parliament, but had kept to local politics'. Winnicott was to be often wilfully modest in his writings, and despite the broad and idiosyncratic range of his references – Keats, W. H. Davies, Foucault, Burke, Shakespeare, Graves – he would always have a distrust of, and professional interest in, the notion of intellectuality. In his own writing he quotes his patients more tellingly than he quotes authoritative texts.

The family described themselves as 'Wesleyan Methodists', and Winnicott was still attending Methodist church at Cambridge before the war until he converted, towards the end of his time there, to the Anglican church. Devon, and Plymouth in particular, had a long-standing tradition of Methodism. Winnicott's work can be seen as both continuing and reacting against different strands of the Dissenting tradition, but we don't know enough about the kind of religious atmosphere in which he grew up to make more than speculative assumptions. He wrote, though, in the plain language that Wesley himself describes in the Preface to his Sermons:

> I design plain truth for plain people: therefore, of set
> purpose, I abstain from all nice and philosophical spec-
> ulations; from all perplexed and intricate reasonings;
> and, as far as possible, from even the show of learning,
> unless in sometimes citing the original Scripture. I
> labour to avoid all words which are not easy to be
> understood, all which are not used in common life; and,
> in particular, those kinds of technical terms that so
> frequently occur in Bodies of Divinity; those modes of
> speaking which men of reading are intimately
> acquainted with, but which to common people are an
> unknown tongue.[6]

Winnicott, like Wesley, wanted to make his work accessible, though without a manifest wish to convert his audience. He in fact once described it as 'the hallmark of
madness when an adult puts too powerful a claim on the
credulity of others',[7] needing to convert them to a particular
point of view. If for 'the original Scripture' in Wesley's
Preface we read 'Freud', and for 'Bodies of Divinity' we read
simply 'psychoanalytic writing' we get something approach-
ing Winnicott's own set purpose. He could make his work
available to a wide range of people without assuming that
popularizing it in some way diminished it. He found the act
of adapting himself to various audiences – like the mother
adapting herself to her infant – productive in itself. 'For
every one lecture', Masud Khan wrote, 'that Winnicott was
asked to give to one of the so-called learned professional
societies, he gave at least a dozen to gatherings of social
workers, child-care organizations, teachers, priests, etc.'[8]
There was an official Winnicott who would be for ever
juggling professional languages and allegiances in front of
learned societies, and a more informal Winnicott who
would say the more plainly outrageous things. In 1936, for
example, in a lecture he gave in Hull, he suggested that

there was 'not so much difference in intellectual capacity at the different ages, only the language and the subjects that engage attention change with the years'.[9] He would also enjoy playing off a language of common-sense against a language of professional expertise. In 1970, in a talk he gave to Anglican priests, he was asked how he would tell whether a person needed psychiatric help. 'If a person comes and talks to you,' he said, 'and, listening to him, you feel he is boring you, then he is sick and needs psychiatric treatment. But if he sustains your interest, no matter how grave his distress or conflict, then you can help him all right.'[10] There is a commitment here, unheard of in psychoanalysis, to affinity between people rather than to a technique of professional help. Winnicott's almost religious commitment to an idea of simple and personal truth, to an ordinary-language psychoanalysis, was inevitably to make his institutional loyalties problematic. It is, of course, the individual's inner conviction that is integral to Nonconformism. Winnicott was to be fiercely and subtly protective of his own difference, as though he was somehow fearful of being seduced by other people's ideas.

In a revealing anecdote from his autobiographical notebook he relates that his father 'had a simple (religious) faith and once when I asked him a question that could have involved us in a long argument he just said: read the Bible and what you find there will be the true answer for you. So I was left, thank God, to get on with it myself.' But the God he thanks here in his droll way, the father who leaves him to the book, could, in Winnicott's various accounts of him, be seen as severe and belittling in his attitude to his son. It is, though, a not unusual family scenario that Winnicott reconstructs. 'When (at twelve years) I one day came home to midday dinner and said "drat" my father looked pained as only he could look, blamed my mother for not seeing to it that I had decent friends, and from that moment he

25

prepared himself to send me away to boarding-school, which he did when I was thirteen. "Drat" sounds very small as a swear word, but he was right; the boy who was my new friend was no good, and he and I could have got into trouble if left to our own devices.' What is striking about these incidents from the autobiographical notebook, apart from the representation of the father as the one who dismisses the son, is Winnicott's seemingly compliant justification of his father's behaviour, as though his conformism was really all for the best. Constituted, as they must be, by the disguised conflicts of retrospective desire, Winnicott's memories of his father are suspiciously cheerful.

The father who is a relatively bland figure in Winnicott's developmental theory, was in Winnicott's account of his early life a potent and potentially humiliating presence. Winnicott describes, in an evocatively contrived scene in the garden of his family home, the upper-middle-class English idyll of his childhood, and its violation:

> Now that slope up from the croquet lawn to the flat part where there is a pond and where there was once a huge clump of pampas grass between the weeping ash trees (by the way do you know what exciting noises the pampas grass makes on a hot Sunday afternoon, when people are lying out on rugs beside the pond, reading or snoozing?). That slope is fraught, as people say, fraught with history. It was on that slope that I took my own private croquet mallet (handle about a foot long because I was only three years old) and I bashed flat the nose of the wax doll that belonged to my sisters and that had become a source of irritation in my life because it was over that doll that my father used to tease me. She was called Rosie. Parodying some popular song he used to say (taunting me by the voice he used)

> Rosie said to Donald
> I love you
> Donald said to Rosie
> I don't believe you do.

(Maybe the verses were the other way round, I forget.) So I knew the doll had to be altered for the worse, and much of my life has been founded on the undoubted fact that I actually did this deed, not merely wished it and planned it.

I was perhaps somewhat relieved when my father took a series of matches and, warming up the wax nose enough, remoulded it so that the face once more became a face. This early demonstration of the restitutive and reparative act certainly made an impression on me, and perhaps made me able to accept the fact that I myself, dear innocent child, had actually become violent directly with a doll, but indirectly with my good-tempered father who was just then entering my conscious life.

Again Winnicott takes a determinedly benign view of his father. The unconvincingly tentative account of what he gained from the experience ('perhaps . . . perhaps . . .') is offset by the strong sense that it was his father who had made the doll problematic for him. Winnicott interprets the incident too narrowly as a displaced Oedipal attack on his father. Despite the teasing and taunting that he obviously felt sensitive to, he does not comment on his father's threat to his masculinity. His possible and ordinary confusion, as a child, about his sexual identity is temporarily resolved by a violent but paradoxical act in which it could not have been clear to him what it was that he was actually trying to destroy. In his developmental theory Winnicott will tell us much about the self as constituted in aggressive assertion, while telling us surprisingly little about what it might be to

27

be a man, or even a woman except in her capacity as a mother.

But it was as 'in a sense . . . an only child with multiple mothers' – which included, in his family, not only two older sisters but also a nanny and governess – that Winnicott chose to remember himself. His father is remembered as letting him down: 'My father was there to kill and be killed, but it is probably true that in the early years he left me too much to all my mothers. Things never quite righted themselves.' In his theoretical work, as we shall see, he would abandon the father and replace him with a fascination for the child and its mothers. It is not the father that interests Winnicott as coming between the mother and child to separate them, but a transitional space from which the father is virtually absent and 'which initially both joins and separates the baby and the mother'.[11] In one of his finest papers, 'The Capacity to be Alone' (1958),[12] Winnicott would suggest that the capacity to be alone depended on, and began with, the child's experience of being alone in the presence of his mother. Because the mother is there, but undemanding (as an auxiliary ego), she can be absent from the child's mind as a total preoccupation; he is safe enough then to lose himself. But Winnicott does not mention, even by implication, the equally significant experience of being alone in the presence of the father. Though, in a sense, relatively free of the father, the child as conceived of in Winnicott's theory was then subject to the potentially disabling pressure of the mother's demand.

Ironically, Winnicott's mother is a more shadowy figure. The few available descriptions of her by his second wife Clare, and other friends, are notably idealized, and therefore improbable and vague: 'vivacious and outgoing . . . able to show and express her feelings easily', 'very friendly and warm-hearted', and so on. Winnicott himself published nothing of note about his mother, but at the age of sixty-

seven he wrote a poem about her which he sent to his
brother-in-law, James Britton, with the words: 'Do you
mind seeing this that hurt coming out of me. I think it had
some thorns sticking out somehow. It's not happened to me
before & I hope it doesn't again.' Before Winnicott went to
boarding school he would do his homework in a special tree
in the garden. The poem, which is called 'The Tree',
includes the following lines:

> Mother below is weeping
>   weeping
>   weeping
> Thus I knew her
>
> Once, stretched out on her lap
>   as now on dead tree
> I learned to make her smile
>   to stem her tears
>   to undo her guilt
>   to cure her inward death
> To enliven her was my living.[13]

In the poem Winnicott clearly identifies himself with
Christ, and the Tree of the title is the Cross. Towards the
end of his life Winnicott became interested in Robert
Graves's novel *King Jesus* and corresponded with Graves
about it. In the novel, which was originally published in
1946, Christ is the man who dedicates himself to being the
zealous enemy of Woman and by doing so becomes one of
her heroes. This, of course, is an irony that could have
appealed to Winnicott for a number of reasons, some of
which will become clear by the end of this book. But in his
poem it is possible that Winnicott was recalling an early
experience of his mother's depression, and her consequent
inability to hold him. The chilling image of himself
'stretched out on her lap/as now on dead tree', by omitting
the definite article suggests that once it is dead it is no tree

in particular, as anonymous as dead wood (Woods, incidentally, was his mother's maiden name). The poem speaks of the absence of what became, in Winnicott's developmental theory, the formative experience in the child's life; the way the mother, in the fullest sense, 'holds' the child, which includes the way the child is held in the mother's mind as well as in her arms. The infant's first environment, in Winnicott's terms, is the experience of being held. It begins before birth and covers the early maternal care that makes possible the infant's psychosomatic integration. 'It took a long time', he wrote, 'for the analytic world . . . to look, for example, at the importance of the way a baby is held; and yet, when you come to think of it, this is of primary significance . . . the question of holding and handling brings up the whole issue of human reliability.'[14]

The poem also alludes to another of Winnicott's central preoccupations as a clinician; the way children attempt to deal with the mother's absence, an absence which can be constituted by her presence in a depressed or otherwise withdrawn mood in which the quality of her attention is unreliable. A child with a seriously depressed mother could, Winnicott wrote, 'feel infinitely dropped'.[15] He would describe in vivid terms infants and young children who had been distracted from their own development by the need to 'look after mother's mood'. A child could feel compelled to enliven an inaccessible mother at the cost of his own spontaneous vitality. He might, as the poem suggests, have to make a living out of keeping his mother alive.

The relatively secure, and perhaps sometimes to his mind overseductive, happiness of his family life made the boarding school he went to in 1910 an exciting opportunity for Winnicott. He could perform himself in new ways. At the Leys School in Cambridge, over two hundred and fifty miles from Plymouth, he was, in his wife's account, 'in his element. To his great delight the afternoons were free, and he ran, cycled, and swam, played rugger, joined the school scouts, and made friends and sang in the choir, and each night he read a story aloud to the boys in his dormitory. He read extremely well and years later I was to benefit from this accomplishment because we were never without a book that he was reading aloud to me . . . He read in a dramatic way, savouring the writing to the full.' In his own writing Winnicott would occasionally make psychoanalysis sound curiously like entertainment. He sometimes found it difficult to keep the language of performance – routine, timing, play, setting and so on – out of his theoretical discourse, and the figure of the actor crops up consistently in his work as an awkward presence. He was apparently to say on more than one occasion that if he hadn't been a psychoanalyst he would like to have been a comic-turn in a music-hall; and his work, in a sense, initiates a comic tradition in psychoanalysis.

It was an interruption in his otherwise busy school life that consolidated his wish to be a doctor. He had broken his collar-bone playing rugby and was in the school sanatorium: 'I could see that for the rest of my life I should have to depend on doctors if I damaged myself or became ill, and the only way out of this position was to become a doctor myself, and from then on the idea as a real proposition was always on my mind, although I know that father expected me to enter his flourishing business and eventually take over from him.' His body and his father posed a threat to the independence he equated at this point in his life with self-sufficiency. In his adolescence Winnicott clearly felt, at least in retrospect, that becoming a doctor, like becoming himself, was some kind of vocation. Allowed by his father, finally, to read medicine, Winnicott was, as he wrote to his friend Stanley Ede at the age of sixteen, 'so excited that all the stored-up feelings about doctors which I have bottled up for so many years seemed to burst and bubble up at once.

31

Do you know that – in the degree that Algy [a shared school friend] wanted to go into a monastery – I have for ever so long wanted to be a doctor. But I have always been afraid that my father did not want it, and so I have never mentioned it and – like Algy – even felt a repulsion at the thought.'[16]

After considerable conflict with his father over the family business, his preference in some sense a betrayal, Winnicott went to Jesus College, Cambridge, in 1914 to read medicine. At the time this involved taking part 1 of the Natural Sciences Tripos (in which Winnicott gained a third class) which then qualified the prospective medical student for the BA degree. He studied, in a Natural Sciences Tripos heavily influenced by Darwin, biology, zoology, comparative anatomy, human anatomy and physiology. In a talk given over forty years later to the Society for Psychosomatic Research he claimed that he was troubled, even then, by the kind of limitations inherent in the version of scientific method he was taught.

The physiology I learned was cold, that is to say, it could be checked up by careful examination of a pithed frog or a heart lung preparation. Every effort was made to eliminate variables such as emotions, and the animals as well as human beings seemed to me to be treated as if they were always in a neutral condition in regard to instinctual life. One can see the civilizing process which brings a dog into a constant state of frustration. Consider the strain that we impose on a dog that does not even secrete urine into the bladder until some indication is given that there will be opportunity for bladder discharge. How much more important it must be that we shall allow physiology to become complicated by emotion and emotional conflict when we study the way the human body works.[17]

With the invention of psychoanalysis Freud was, in a sense, to 'allow physiology to become complicated by emotion', but he wrote very little about feelings, about the emotions themselves, referring instead to what were called in the Standard Edition translation 'affects', and these were conceived of as representations of instinctual derivatives. As a result psychoanalysis in England inherited an impoverished affective vocabulary. What Winnicott here calls the 'variables' in the science he was taught became the focus of study in the version of psychoanalysis that Winnicott practised. In Winnicott's work emotion as interference with the data was to be replaced by enquiry into what could interfere with emotional development. The obstacles, for both analyst and patient, were revealed to be the instruments. As a medical doctor who became a psychoanalyst, Winnicott was always to experience a divided duty. 'I absolutely believe', he wrote, 'in objectivity and in looking at things straight and doing things about them; but not in making it boring by forgetting the fantasy, the unconscious fantasy.'[18] It was not science *per se* that was reductive, but any method that made things boring. To be boring, Winnicott implies here, is somehow to trivialize: and unconscious fantasy was what made things interesting. He was to be interested, in his early theoretical work, in what happened to the scientific pragmatist when he allowed himself the idea of an unconscious.

Winnicott's years as a medical student in Cambridge were disrupted by the war. Described by a friend as 'a medical student who liked to sing a comic song on Saturday evenings in the ward – and sang "Apple Dumplings" and cheered us all up', Winnicott worked in the colleges that were turned into military hospitals. As a medical student he was exempt from the army, and the loss of so many of his friends killed in the war was to be one of the haunting regrets of his life.

Eventually, in 1917, Winnicott was accepted as a Surgeon

Probationer on a destroyer. He was one of the youngest men aboard and the only Medical Officer, so he had considerable responsibility. The ship was involved in some enemy action, but in his brief experience which lasted till the end of the war he had, according to his wife, 'much free time which he seems to have spent reading the novels of Henry James'. Despite the casual irony of her account, the information about Winnicott's reading is an appropriate antidote to Winnicott's own peculiar kind of disclaimed sophistication (James, of course, like Winnicott, was preoccupied in his novels by what was elusively absent). But it was clearly very important to Winnicott to have participated in some way, to have, in his phrase, 'contributed in'. His early adulthood, like his early middle age, was dominated by a world war. They were to be, in different ways, inevitably crucial experiences in what would otherwise have been decisive developmental stages in his life.

In 1918, at the end of the war, Winnicott went to St Bartholomew's Hospital in London to finish his medical training. It seems that he either never took, or certainly never passed, his third MB in surgery, midwifery and gynaecology, but by 1920 he was a qualified doctor specializing in what was then called children's medicine. He had always shared with his sisters what was regarded as a family talent for getting on with children, and throughout his training he had been interested in children's problems ('Donald Winnicott had the most astonishing powers with children,' his colleague the paediatrician Jack Tizard wrote in his obituary of Winnicott. 'To say that he understood children would to me sound false and vaguely patronizing: it was rather that children understood him . . .'[19]). Winnicott had originally wanted to be a General Medical Practitioner somewhere in the country, and the idea of being a country doctor at that time still had a romance of its own. He was a familiar and reassuringly heroic figure in the great nineteenth-century

English novels that Winnicott read so keenly. But in 1919 a friend lent him Freud's *Interpretation of Dreams* – it had first been translated in 1913 by A. A. Brill – and the book clearly made a powerful impression on him. He wrote a letter of almost visionary enthusiasm to his sister Violet explaining psychoanalysis:

> I am putting all this extremely simply. If there is anything which is not completely simple for anyone to understand I want you to tell me because I am now practising so that one day I will be able to introduce the subject to English people so that who runs may read.[20]

At the age of twenty-three, and prompted by reading Freud, Winnicott had found a new vocation in addition to medicine: it was to make available the difficult (or the repressed) by a process of 'simple' redescription. But it is of interest in the light of Winnicott's relationship with Freud that reference to the *Interpretation of Dreams* itself turns up for the first time in the books published during his lifetime in a footnote to his last book, *Playing and Reality*. And it is not listed in the bibliographies of his two main volumes of collected papers (Winnicott 1958 and 1965).

Winnicott would often be at his most revealing in his summarizing accounts, of which there are many, of Freud's contribution and its bearing on his own work:

> The reader should know that I am a product of the Freudian or psychoanalytic school. This does not mean that I take for granted everything Freud said or wrote, and in any case that would be absurd since Freud was developing, that is to say changing, his views (in an orderly manner, like any other scientific worker) all along the line right up to his death in 1939.
>
> As a matter of fact, there are some things that Freud came to believe which seem to me and to many other

35

analysts to be actually wrong, but it simply does not matter. The point is that Freud started off a scientific approach to the problem of human development; he broke through the reluctance to speak openly of sex and especially of infant and child sexuality, and he accepted the instincts as basic and worthy of study; he gave us a method for use and for development which we could learn, and whereby we could check the observations of others and contribute our own; he demonstrated the repressed unconscious and the operation of unconscious conflict; he insisted on the full recognition of psychic reality (what is real to the individual apart from what is actual); he boldly attempted to formulate theories of the mental processes, some of which have already become generally accepted.[21]

Winnicott is edgy, as ever, about his allegiances. Brackets are used characteristically for revisions presented as clarifications, or for reassurance that an implied criticism is not seen as a misrepresentation. Given Winnicott's specific interests, the difference between Freud developing and Freud changing his views would seem to be of some significance. What he is at pains to stress here, though, seems to be the idea which Freud himself was committed to, that Freud was a scientist and that psychoanalysis was a science, albeit a relatively new one. Coming from paediatric medicine to psychoanalysis in his early twenties, Winnicott was to work on the overlap between them. In what sense was Freud 'like any other scientific worker' (a mild disparagement which of course involves the question of Winnicott's transference to Freud)? Both Winnicott's analysts, James Strachey and Joan Rivière, had been analysed by Freud and translated his work. Was it an oversimplification and therefore a denial to suggest, as Winnicott was later to do, that psychoanalysis was an extended history-taking ('Psychoanalysis for me is a vast extension of history-taking, with therapeutics as a by-product'[22])? Winnicott was to enter the British Psychoanalytical Society as the whole issue of lay (non-medical) analysis was being debated. In 1926, the year Melanie Klein first came to London, Freud published his most influential contribution on the subject, *The Question of Lay Analysis*. In 1927 the British Society would form a Sub-committee on Lay Analysis. Neither Anna Freud nor Melanie Klein, the founding mothers of child analysis, were doctors (Klein had wanted to train as a doctor but her family had prevented her[23]). Winnicott was therefore uniquely placed to continue his life-long interest in psychosomatics, intimately bound up as it was with the very puzzling question of what kind of practice psychoanalysis was.

In 1923 Winnicott qualified as a consultant in children's medicine and was appointed to work at the Queen's Hospital for Children in Hackney, where he also ran the London County Council Rheumatic and Heart Clinic, and at Paddington Green Children's Hospital where he was to work for over forty years, and which he would refer to as his 'Psychiatric Snack-Bar' (later, in a similar kind of analogy, Winnicott suggested that a psychoanalyst was like a prostitute, there to be used). In the same year, at the age of twenty-seven, he married Alice Taylor, a potter, and began a ten-year analysis with James Strachey, the man who was to do the standard translation of Freud into English, and who had himself been analysed by Freud. In the obituary for Strachey that Winnicott later wrote – Strachey died in 1969 – he traced a distinctively Winnicottian line of descent:

> I would say that Strachey had one thing quite clear in his mind as a result of his visit to Freud: that a process develops in the patient, and that what transpires cannot be produced but it can be made use of. This is what I feel about my own analysis with Strachey, and in my

work I have tried to follow the principle through and to emphasize the idea in its stark simplicity. It is my experience of analysis at the hand of Strachey that has made me suspicious of descriptions of interpretative work in analysis which seem to give credit to the interpretations for all that happens, as if the process in the patient had got lost sight of.'[24]

As we shall see, in Winnicott's version of psychoanalysis it was the developmental process of the patient that determined the analysis. Interpretation simply facilitated this process, it could not usurp it, except at the cost of the patient's true self. His interest in infancy would feed his scepticism about the role of verbal interpretation in psychoanalytic treatment. Strachey, however, had written his most influential paper on the idea of what he called the 'mutative interpretation' as the crucial instrument of change in psychoanalysis. This Winnicott did not emphasize in the obituary.[25]

In the same year that Winnicott wrote the obituary he was corresponding with someone about his interest in Wycliffe (like Strachey a translator, but of the Bible) and the Lollards, a far more nonconformist sect than the Methodists. 'My feeling is that I am a natural Lollard,' he wrote, 'and would have had a bad time in the 14th and 15th centuries . . . I am even interested in the word Lollard but it would be very complex to describe to you in one letter how this comes in in connection with my work . . .'[26] The Lollards were fourteenth-century heretics, either actual followers of Wycliffe or supporters of some of his views. The word Lollard means an idler, mutterer or droner, from *lollen* meaning 'to mew, bawl, or mutter'. In 1923 Winnicott started in the interpretative discipline of psychoanalysis, as a doctor with a special interest in the process of development, and in those who mew, bawl and eventually begin to mutter.

2 History-taking

'Why,' said the Dodo, 'the best way to
explain it is to do it.'
Lewis Carroll

I THE BRITISH SOCIETY

In 1913 Ernest Jones, the leading British psychoanalyst,
founded the London Psychoanalytical Society. There were
fifteen members and only four practising analysts. Transla-
tions of Freud's work into English were gradually becoming
available, but the only experienced analysts were working
in Vienna (Freud and his immediate circle), Berlin (Abraham) and Budapest (Ferenczi). German was the shared
psychoanalytic language. So when Jones dissolved the
London Society after the war and set up the British Psycho-
analytical Society in 1919, it was, in the fullest sense, an
act of courageous translation. Psychoanalysis was a new
German, and for some, Jewish, science and was subjected to
suspicious scrutiny, particularly by the British Medical
Association. The first ten years of the new Society were
immensely productive, partly because of the opposition and
incomprehension psychoanalysis met with in London. By
the time Winnicott began his analysis with James Strachey
in 1923 they had organized and published the *International
Journal of Psycho-Analysis* (1920), which Strachey himself
edited, founded the *British Journal of Medical Psychology*
through the pressure of the analysts in the British Psychological Society (1920), and started the International Psycho-

39

Analytical Library (1921), edited by Ernest Jones and published by the Hogarth Press which was owned by Leonard and Virginia Woolf. By 1930 there was an Institute of Psycho-Analysis (1924), a London Clinic of Psycho-Analysis (1926), and the Eleventh International Psycho-Analytical Congress – which Freud did not attend – had been held in Oxford (1929).[1]

But in the first ten years of its existence the Society had to face two overriding, related issues. First, there was the question of lay analysis, of whether psychoanalysis should be conceived of as a branch of medicine, a science only to be practised by doctors. And secondly, prompted largely by the arrival of Melanie Klein in London in 1926, the new question of child analysis, of its legitimacy as a branch of psychoanalysis. It began to seem that advances in psycho-analytic theory might increasingly come from child analysts, and yet Anna Freud and Melanie Klein, who had virtually founded the new discipline, were both lay analysts. As a paediatrician training to be a psychoanalyst, and beginning to practise child analysis himself, Winnicott was in a unique position in the British Society. He played an essential part in what he would later call – referring to his concept of the transitional object – 'the interplay between separateness and union'[2] of the various groups that were to emerge in the British Society.

But in its early days the British Society was keen to ally itself with the recognized and respectable medical profession. Despite the fact that in 1927, according to Ernest Jones, 40 per cent of the Society were lay analysts, the Abbreviated Report of the Sub-committee on Lay Analysis concluded, '. . . the British Psychoanalytical Society is practically unanimously of the opinion that most analysts should be medical but that a proportion of lay analysts should be freely admitted provided that certain conditions are fulfilled.' So when Winnicott's analyst James Strachey,

Lytton Strachey's brother, had approached Jones about training to be an analyst he had been advised to start a medical
training. He entered St Thomas's Hospital but lasted only
three weeks. Before he began his analysis with Freud he
had, in his own words, 'a discreditable academic career with
the barest of BA degrees, no medical qualifications, no
knowledge of the physical sciences, no experience of any-
thiing except third-rate journalism. The only thing in my
favour was that at the age of thirty I wrote a letter out of
the blue to Freud, asking him if he would take me on as a
student.'³ Commenting on Strachey's involvement in psychoanalysis, Perry Meisel has written that in England,
unlike the rest of Europe, 'psychoanalysis lingered longer in
a state of generous dilettantism; as nonmedical practition-
ers, James and Alix (his wife) were rather unusual because
they made it the principal focus of their lives. Anthropolo-
gists, art historians, economists, as well as doctors of
various persuasions – even literary types like Lytton –
dabbled in psychoanalysis, seeing it as a contribution to
their chosen specialties, not a profession in itself. As a
result, the British interest in psychoanalysis was strikingly
diverse.'⁴ Winnicott saw psychoanalysis as contributing in
a crucial way to his chosen speciality of paediatrics. A
qualified doctor, he began his own analysis as one of the
first two patients of a relatively untrained lay analyst, who
was also to become an important member of a British
Society not well disposed to non-medical analysts.

Soon after Winnicott began his analysis, Alix Strachey
went to be analysed by Karl Abraham in Berlin where she
met and became friendly with Melanie Klein. Klein had also
begun an analysis with Abraham in 1924, having previously
been analysed in Budapest by Ferenczi. By this time Klein
and Freud's daughter Anna were emerging as the inaugur-
ators of the new, and in some ways more shocking, discipline of the psychoanalysis of children. Alix Strachey

translated Klein's early papers on child analysis, and they aroused considerable interest and controversy in London. In July 1925, the year Winnicott's mother died, Klein gave a series of six lectures on child analysis to the British Society in London. At Christmas of the same year Abraham died, so in 1926 Ernest Jones, who had always been a keen supporter of Klein's work, invited her to come to London, where she lived until her death in 1960. Though not everyone found her work inspiring – Edward Glover described it in a famous critique as 'merely a matriarchal variant of the doctrine of Original Sin'⁵ – she certainly found London a sympathetic environment for her work, quickly establishing herself as a pioneer in the British Society, with devoted followers and critics.

By 1927 both Melanie Klein and Anna Freud had conducted several extensive analyses of children and could bring to bear on psychoanalytic theory their new kind of clinical experience. There were, however, considerable differences between them. While Anna Freud largely endorsed her father's views, Klein's work provided a new way of looking at the development of the young pre-Oedipal child. In 1927 Anna Freud published her book on the technique of child analysis, *Einfuhrung in die Technik der Kinderanalyse* – which, significantly, was not translated until 1946. It prompted a debate in the British Society about the relative merits of Anna Freud's and Klein's approaches to child analysis. This debate, the 'Symposium on Child Analysis', Winnicott could not attend because he was not a full member of the Society. But the discussion concerning the new rival psychoanalytic discourses on the child became an important backdrop to his work.

There were three main points of disagreement between Anna Freud and Klein, all derived from Klein's growing sense of an early and complex internal world of fantasy that even the very young child was able to represent through play, and which the analyst could interpret along classical lines. First, Klein was critical of the 'elaborate and troublesome means' Anna Freud prescribed, in the initial period of the treatment, to gain the child's confidence. To cultivate a positive transference only colluded, in her view, with the child's denial of his most unacceptable, hostile feelings. Secondly, Klein's 'play-technique' of child analysis, in which the child was offered a small number of simple toys with which to represent his fantasy life, had revealed all the structures Freud had described in the Oedipal child (Ego, Id and Super-Ego) but in much younger children, and in more primitive forms. In Anna Freud's view the pre-Oedipal child did not have a sufficiently developed Ego to be able to free-associate. And since the Super-Ego (the paternal prohibition on incestuous desire which the child internalizes) was, as Freud had written, the 'heir of the Oedipus Complex', the pre-Oedipal child could have no firmly established internal controls of his own erotic and aggressive impulses. This meant that for Anna Freud the child analyst was less an interpreter of unconscious conflict in the child, than an exemplary adult with whom the child could identify as part of his education in self-control. So Klein's third major criticism of Anna Freud's clinical technique was that if the analyst was both educator and object of emulation the child would no longer be free to represent to the analyst what he was feeling. In Klein's view Anna Freud was using a crude form of analytic technique to teach the child impulse control, while she favoured a slightly modified version of the classical technique to explore the meaning of, and gain access to, the child's deepest feelings.

Joan Rivière, a devoted follower of Klein who was to be Winnicott's second analyst, summed up the Kleinian position at the Symposium by stating that psychoanalysis was 'not concerned with the real world, nor with the child's or adult's adaptation to the real world, nor with sickness nor

health, nor virtue nor vice. It is concerned simply and solely
with the imaginings of the childish mind, the phantasied
pleasures and the dreaded retributions.'[6] There is the smug-
ness of excessive rigour in this, but Klein, by narrowing her
focus, had intensified her conviction, and the conviction of
her followers. The child's internal world, as recreated in the
analytic situation, had become, by a kind of psychoanalytic
refinement, a sufficient context in which to understand the
child.

Winnicott was to take as seriously as Anna Freud did the
importance of the child's actual parents – whose help he
would often enlist in the treatment – and the circumstances
in which they lived. Klein, for example, makes little reference in her work to social or economic conditions. Also,
like Anna Freud, Winnicott would be less strictly non-
collusive with the child than Klein had advised. But it was
to Klein's theory that Winnicott naturally gravitated. From
his experience in paediatrics ('At that time no other analyst
was also a paediatrician so for two or three decades I was an
isolated phenomenon'[7]) he came to Klein's work with his
own conviction about the significance for development of
the pre-Oedipal period in the child's life. He recalled in
1962:

> At that time, in the 1920s, everything had the Oedipus
> complex at its core. The analysis of the psycho-neuroses
> led the analyst over and over again to the anxieties
> belonging to the instinctual life at the four- to five-year
> period in the child's relationship to the two parents.
> Earlier difficulties that came to light were treated in
> analyses as regressions to pre-genital fixation points,
> but the dynamics came from conflict at the full-blown
> genital Oedipus complex of the toddler or late toddler
> age, that is just before the passing of the Oedipus
> complex and the onset of the latency period. Now,

innumerable case histories showed me that the children who became disturbed, whether psycho-neurotic, psychotic, psycho-somatic or anti-social, showed difficulties in their emotional development in infancy, even as babies. Paranoid hypersensitive children could even have started to be in that pattern in the first weeks or even days of life. Something was wrong somewhere. When I came to treat children by psycho-analysis I was able to confirm the origin of psycho-neurosis in the Oedipus complex, and yet I knew that troubles started earlier.[8]

When Strachey, as Winnicott put it, 'broke into his analysis of me and told me about Melanie Klein' – an intervention which led to his being supervised by her – he was fascinated by 'the immense amount that I found she knew already', but at the same time troubled. It was as though he felt slightly outraged at her intrusion into what he must have regarded as his own territory. 'This was difficult for me,' he wrote, 'because overnight I had changed from being a pioneer into being a student with a pioneer teacher':[9] wherever he went, he met a woman on her way back. As an experienced paediatrician but a student psychoanalyst Winnicott had to struggle in his late twenties to maintain a position of his own. In a passing reference to Klein's conflict with Anna Freud in this same paper Winnicott points out his own position by appearing to take a side. For Klein, he writes, 'child analysis was exactly like adult analysis. This was never a trouble from my point of view as I started with the same view, and I hold this view now. The idea of a preparatory period belongs to the type of case, not to a set technique belonging to child analysis.'[10] Where Klein had said that a preparatory period in child analysis was intrinsically misleading, and Anna Freud had said that it was indispensable to the treatment, Winnicott, supposedly agreeing with Klein, suggests that it always depended on the case. He would argue that technique, to be of any value, had to be adapted to the individual patient. The idea of technique in analysis, by the generalization it implied, was a denial of the differences between people. 'I do adapt quite a little', he wrote, 'to individual expectations at the very beginning. It is unhuman not to do so.'[11] It was often Winnicott's inclination to dispel a contradiction, here between Klein and Anna Freud, with a paradox. To find a third position that would combine, and so modify, two apparently incompatible options.[12]

Though Winnicott would describe Klein, in 1959, as representing 'the most vigorous attempt to study the earliest processes of the developing human infant apart from the study of child-care',[13] he found much of what she had to teach him compatible, at first, with what he himself had discovered. He particularly valued in the earliest stages of their professional relationship her 'way of making inner psychic reality very real',[14] but he would increasingly distrust the opposing dogmas in child analysis. 'It is clear that this dichotomy', he wrote, 'between those who almost confine their researches to a study of the internal processes and those who are interested in infant care is a temporary dichotomy in psychoanalytic discussion, one which will eventually disappear by natural processes.'[15] Winnicott's belief in natural processes turned out, in this case, to be wishful thinking. But in the late 1920s, when this dichotomy first became an issue in psychoanalysis, Winnicott learned from Klein something about the child's internal world that was to be crucial to his own development.

But having worked out the basic constituents of the child's internal world, the risk for the Kleinian analyst was of seeming to know beforehand all there was to know about the child. Klein's apparently comprehensive knowledge of the child's unconscious could be used as a blueprint. From the very beginning Winnicott would represent himself as less knowing than Klein as an analyst; and he would stress the importance, as an analyst, of being able to tolerate not-knowing. Klein had described the child's wish for knowledge – what she called the 'epistemophilic instinct' – as integral to his development, and this led her to overvalue the insight gained from interpretation in analysis. Winnicott would never insist on Klein's equation of development and the acquisition of knowledge. And in his later work he would replace the capacity to know by the capacity to play, as a criterion for health. In Winnicott's work it would sometimes seem as though for him the (perhaps unconscious) aim of any method, or set of rules, was to make possible new kinds of anomalies. He would, as we shall see, take from Klein what he wanted without becoming either a devotee or a connoisseur of her theory. 'I do not claim', he wrote in 1962, 'to be able to hand out the Klein view in a way that she would herself approve of. I believe my views began to separate out from hers, and in any case I found she had not included me in as a Kleinian. This did not matter to me because I have never been able to follow anyone else, not even Freud. But Freud was easy to criticize, because he was always critical of himself.'[16]

There is clearly some bitterness in this retrospective view. Between 1935 and 1939 Winnicott was to psychoanalyse Klein's son, Eric, though without acceding to her demand that she supervise the case. And Melanie Klein was to analyse Winnicott's second wife Clare. It was a passionate and troubled life-long involvement. But in the 1930s, supervised by Klein, and in a second analysis (1933–8) with Joan Rivière, Winnicott came to the making of psychoanalytic theory with equally strong but less strident ideas of his own about the treatment of children.

II WINNICOTT: THE PAEDIATRICIAN AS ANALYST

Aware of the unwillingness of the medical profession to 'recognize the unconscious, and to admit the importance and intensity of childish erotism and hostility',[17] Winnicott set out in his early papers and first book, *Clinical Notes on Disorders of Childhood* (1931), a new approach for doctors to the treatment of ordinary childhood problems. His belief in the importance of children's feelings, and the insights made possible by psychoanalysis, had made him critical of contemporary medical attitudes to children's symptoms. The unconscious, as described by Freud and Klein, had to be admitted, owned up to and allowed in. But not, he was keen to add, at the cost of an empirical approach to paediatrics. 'The truth is', he wrote, 'that my point of view is obvious to anyone who makes for himself opportunity for the observation of the working of children's feelings.'[18] It was, however, 'necessary to point out how much more intense the infant's feelings are than one can tell through empathy'.[19] For the adult, and for his medical colleagues, estranged from the intensity of the most primitive infantile feelings Klein had described, it could seem like an act of rash inference, and even blind faith, to take such childish feelings seriously. 'In all ages', as Winnicott wrote, 'there are the few who believe in the little child's feelings, and the majority who deny or sentimentalize.'[20] And there were perhaps also cultural factors at work in the relative insensitivity of the British doctor to children's feelings. The original psychoanalysts, and Klein herself, were not English, and their experience of recent history was of course quite different. 'The Englishman', Winnicott wrote, '. . . does not want to be upset, to be reminded that there are personal tragedies all over the place, that he is not really happy himself; in short – he refuses to be put off his golf.'[21] Clinically, he had taken his lead, as he would write in the

Introduction to *Playing and Reality*, from 'the descriptions that parents are able to give of their experiences with their children if we know how to give them the chance to remember in their own way and time'.[22] He was beginning to define, in his earliest work, a new kind of competence in which treatment was the provision of an opportunity for the patient, an opportunity to make himself known.

Being a psychoanalyst as well as a paediatrician had, he wrote, 'increased [his] natural tendency to be interested in the person, the personality rather than in tissues as such, or in diseases'.[23] But as a scientist writing for what was then a predominantly medical audience, Winnicott was keen to square his unconventional approach – seeing symptoms as the expression of feelings – with a version of biology:

> The theory which explains these symptoms by giving to emotional confict the respect due to it is not only capable of proof in individual cases, but is also satisfactory biologically. These symptoms are typically human and the great difference between the human being and other mammals is, perhaps, the much more complicated attempt on the part of the former to make the instincts serve instead of govern. And in this attempt is naturally to be sought the causes of the illnesses which are common in man and practically absent in animals.[24]

Man is characterized here by what makes him ill, his wish for mastery over his instinctual life. He suffers, as Freud had suggested, from the attitudes he is compelled to take towards his instincts. From the psychoanalytic perspective that Winnicott used to describe the child's symptoms, shyness, enuresis, fidgetiness, eczema were no longer a physiological malfunction, but intelligent and therefore intelligible solutions to emotional conflict. 'Typically human', these common childhood symptoms were not isolated anomalies in the child's development but integral to the child's life. In

Bed-wet

49

the full context of the child's life, of 'the feelings of the whole person, his place in his environment, and the emotional state of his whole personality',[25] the symptom emerges as a viable form of self-cure for the child. 'The movements of the anxious child', for example, Winnicott suggests, 'are part of the child's effort to master anxiety.'[26]

It is not the symptom, Winnicott proposes, but the child's use of the symptom that can be pathological. 'Abnormality', he writes, 'shows in a limitation and a rigidity in the child's capacity to employ symptoms, and a relative lack of relationship between the symptoms.'[27] He offers bed-wetting as a common example: 'If by bed-wetting the child is making effective protest against strict management, sticking up for the rights of the individual, so to speak, then the symptom is not an illness; rather it is a sign that the child still hopes to keep the individuality which has been in some way threatened.'[28] Symptoms become rigidified, habitual, and part of an illness pattern when they are ineffective as communications, when they fail to protect the child's development. Symptoms are part of the way the child works on and through his inevitable difficulties in living; the healthy child has a flexible repertoire of symptoms, that work as communications to the environment. 'It is these devices', Winnicott writes,

> that are normally employed by our children that we call symptoms, and we say that a normal child is able to have any kind of symptom in appropriate circumstances. But with an ill child it is not the symptoms that are the trouble; it is the fact that the symptoms are not doing their job, and are as much a nuisance to the child as to the mother.

> So although bed-wetting, and refusal of food, and all sorts of other symptoms can be serious indications for treatment, they need not be so. In fact, children who

can surely be called normal can be shown to have such
symptoms, and to have them simply because life is
difficult, inherently difficult for every human being, for
every one from the very beginning.[29]

What is repressed in the symptom is the context that makes
it intelligible. Taking an accurate history, something which
Klein mentions infrequently in her work, was for Winnicott
virtually synonymous with both diagnosis and treatment:

> The doctor gets from the parents as clear a picture as he
> can of the child's past life, and of his present state, and
> he tries to relate the symptoms for which the child is
> brought to the child's personality, and to his external
> and internal experiences.[30]

The 'lack of history-taking' in which 'no one has troubled
to seek out these facts or to string them together' isolates
the child from the sense of his symptom. Winnicott's image
is too familiar to be immediately striking; the details of a
child's life might be like beads that are all over the place
waiting to be strung together, and they can of course be
strung together in a variety of ways. The analyst helps
gather them for the patient and they string things together.
Over twenty years later Winnicott would write a fascinat-
ing, brief paper, out of a different but related context,
entitled, 'String: a Technique of Communication'(1960).[31]
   In the glimpses of her clinical work that Klein offered in
her early papers she recommended continual interpretation
of the children's play. She was translating the child's communications along the psychoanalytic lines she had laid
out, and the material needed to be translated because it was
so deeply unacceptable to the child. Winnicott assumed that
the child had a primary wish to be understood, indeed 'longs
for someone to bring understanding'.[32] He does not begin
with the conventional psychoanalytic conviction that the

child is self-evasive. The Winnicottian child tends to be a collaborator rather than an antagonist, so Winnicott's early papers present a less imposing therapeutic presence than Klein's. 'By understanding management of an anxious child,' he writes, 'which usually means inactive observation without anxiety on the part of the doctor, return to health in many cases can be hastened.'[33] The doctor becomes a sympathetic witness to the child's distress, and the doctor's unanxious recognition of the child's predicament, what Winnicott calls elsewhere 'appreciative understanding', is itself an intervention. The doctor is 'meeting need with appropriate action, or studied inaction'.[34] But this modest proposal, which could be seen as the blandest kind of therapeutic quietism, conceals a pointed question: what is the anxiety in the analyst that might make him need to interpret, or the anxiety in the doctor that might make him want to do something more active than listen? Winnicott describes

> an intelligent girl of twelve who had become nervous at school and enuretic at night. No one seemed to have realized that she was struggling with her grief at her favourite brother's death . . . events had taken place in such a way that she never experienced acute grief, and yet grief was there waiting for acknowledgement. I caught her with an unexpected 'You were very fond of him, weren't you?' which produced loss of control, and floods of tears. The result of this was a return to normal at school, and a cessation of the enuresis at night.[35]

Winnicott, of course, is not describing, as Klein was in her early papers, extensive psychoanalytic treatments, nor are the patients he describes as disturbed as hers were. There are still comparisons to be drawn. Clinically, as in this example, Winnicott tends to look, not for what is remotely unconscious, the esoteric unknown, but for what is there in a person 'waiting for acknowledgement'. He 'caught her', as though she was falling, with something simple that she could recognize, but because she was dissociated from her grief, could not have anticipated.

Winnicott describes in these early papers another child of ten called Peggy, for whom

> the parents' taboo of sexual matters had been an important factor in her illness, more important than the unusually complicated nature of the home life she had experienced. Through meeting my attitude toward sexual matters, which was relatively free from anxiety, she was enabled to deal with the material that was already present in her mind. In other words what the child needed, and got, was sexual enlightenment; but I did not directly enlighten her, I only provided a blackboard on which she chalked up her own observations. This could not have been successful in so short a time if she had been a markedly neurotic individual.[36]

From a psychoanalytic perspective the patient is always suffering from the self-knowledge he has had to refuse himself. Winnicott emphasizes in his first psychoanalytic papers that it is an 'attitude . . . relatively free from anxiety', not exclusively the interpretative process which can be a part of that attitude, that enables the child to become intelligible to herself. He does not so much interpret the child's defences as allow for them. He assumes that the child has a wish to make sense to herself, but that she cannot be directly informed of what she already knows. The invitation in the analyst's attitude facilitates her self-representation.

Freud had written that 'the doctor should be opaque to his patients and, like a mirror, should show them nothing but what is shown to him'.[31] For Winnicott the analytic setting would be the provision of a metaphorical blackboard on which the patient chalks up his own observations. 'The principle is', he wrote in *Playing and Reality*, 'that it is the patient and only the patient who has the answers. We may or may not enable him or her to encompass what is known or become aware of it with acceptance.'[38] Taking for granted the child's wish to make himself known, to himself through others, we see Winnicott working in these early papers with the child's opportunism, the child's capacity and willingness to use the environment in the service of the developmental process. His psychoanalytic method is minimal and unobtrusive.

But in one of his earliest papers (never republished), 'Skin Changes in Relation to Emotional Disorder' (1938), Winnicott expressed profound ambivalence about psychoanalysis itself. Advocating that doctors should know about 'the psychology of the unconscious' and its 'mechanisms', he suggests that the older postgraduate doctor, by virtue of his relative maturity, 'should be able to stand a familiarity with these mechanisms without too much loss of spontaneity and intuitive understanding'.[39] Winnicott acknowledges here that an adherence to psychoanalytic theory, to knowledge of the unconscious, might cramp more idiosyncratic kinds of understanding.[40] There was a personal cost to being informed about these mechanisms. For Winnicott health would always be characterized by spontaneity and intuition, ideas which barely figure in Freud or Klein. And he would particularly value 'the feelings of those who do not much like thinking things out. They act best on intuition.'[41] Spontaneity and intuition, of course, cannot be calculated. They are beyond anticipation. To Winnicott, despite the emphasis throughout his work on dependence, any theoretical allegiance ran the risk of becoming a compliant act, of pre-empting the personal and the unexpected. 'It is not possible to be original,' he wrote in *Playing and Reality*, 'except on a basis of tradition.'[42] But a tradition was only useful, in his view, if it provided opportunity for innovation. As we shall see, in his first important psychoanalytic paper, 'The Manic Defence',[43] he expressed his gratitude to Klein through lucid redescription of her work, and explicit confirmation of its value, while including an almost parodic piece of personal dissent.

III THE MANIC DEFENCE AND THE PLACE OF PLEASURE

In 1935 Melanie Klein presented her paper, 'A Contribution to the Psychogenesis of Manic Depressive States',[44] to the British Society. In it she formulated for the first time her concept of a depressive position in development. It was a landmark in her work, and a revision of psychoanalytic theory, because the depressive position replaced, for the Kleinians, the centrality Freud had accorded to the later Oedipus Complex. The Kleinian analysts in the British Society were those who accepted the concept of a depressive position. Winnicott, who never wanted to be considered as a Kleinian analyst, replied at the end of the same year with a paper of his own, entitled 'The Manic Defence'. In this paper, which qualified him for membership of the British Society, he affirmed the value for him of Klein's new insights, which he referred to throughout his later work, while occasionally speaking, as it were, on behalf of the manic defence. Klein had, in her paper, put psychic pain – fear, guilt, anxiety, depression – at the centre of human development. And a lot of ordinary human pleasures were implicitly represented by her as ways of managing, by avoidance, psychic pain. Reacting to Klein sometimes as though she were a tyrannical parent, Winnicott seeks in his paper to answer an endearingly crude question: was it merely part of one's own manic defence, and therefore a confirmation of her theory, to feel that Klein, as represented by her theory, was a bit of a killjoy? Her implied account of what a good life might be did seem to preclude a lot of pleasure, and she seemed quite untroubled by her own conviction. Her paper was, for example, unselfconsciously dense with her own terminology, paying no attention to the medium in which she wrote. Winnicott's paper, packed as it is with references to language, was at least attentive to the fact that psychoanalytic theory, like a person's account of his feelings, is made with words.

Klein's description of the depressive position made it possible to conceive in a new way of the infant's developmental task, and to link infantile states of mind with adult psychosis. For the infant, Klein wrote, 'all depends on how it is able to find its way out of the conflict between love and uncontrollable hatred and sadism'.[45] Up until about six months the infant has desired and attacked and been attached to what Klein refers to as part-objects. From his point of view the mother has been two disparate and unrelated part-objects – an available good-breast that nourishes him and that he loves, and a bad-breast that he destroys and can experience as attacking him in retaliation. He protects the good-breast that he needs from his own destructiveness by the defensive procedures that Klein calls splitting and idealization. He 'splits' the mother into good and bad parts, overprotecting the good part by overvaluing it. The two parts never meet in his mind for fear of the consequences. With the depressive position comes the idea of the mother as a whole person commensurate with but also distinct from the infant's existence. 'When the child comes to know the mother as a whole person', Klein writes, 'and becomes identified with her as a whole, real and loved person ... then the depressive position ... comes to the fore.'[46] The infant at the depressive position has to tolerate the guilt and anxiety that arise from concern about having damaged the person he loves. This involves a full realization of his own destructiveness and its consequences, and so brings with it new defences to deal with a new kind of psychic pain. 'The depressive position', Hanna Segal writes in a concise commentary on Klein's paper,

> mobilizes additional defences of a manic nature. In essence, those defences are directed against experiencing the psychic reality of the depressive pain, and their main characteristic is a denial of psychic reality. Dependence on the object and ambivalence are denied and the object is omnipotently controlled and treated with triumph and contempt so that the loss of the object shall not give rise to pain or guilt. Alternately, or simultaneously, there may be a flight to the idealized internal object, denying any feeling of destruction and loss.[47]

By the use of the manic defence the individual is emotionally impoverished but apparently protected from what is felt to be intolerable pain. He manipulates a fantasy of self-sufficiency to disengage himself from the painful consequences of exchange with real objects, and contact with his own psychic reality. It was to Klein's new topography of psychic reality and its attendant defences that Winnicott was to turn his attention in 'The Manic Defence'. He defined the manic defence itself succinctly in the last sentence of his paper:

> The term manic defence is intended to cover a person's capacity to deny the depressive anxiety that is inherent in emotional development, anxiety that belongs to the capacity of the individual to feel guilt, and also to acknowledge responsibility for instinctual experiences, and for the aggression in the fantasy that goes with instinctual experience.[48]

57

Apart from its clarity, this is unexceptional. It is, however, characteristically Winnicottian. He tends, throughout his work, to write of capacities rather than positions or stages. The emphasis on capacity in his work allows for individual differences. 'Capacity', with its implication of stored possibility, and its combination of the receptive and the generative, blurs the boundary between activity and passivity. It is also characteristic of Winnicott that the final sentence is uncontroversially of a piece with Klein's point of view, when the paper itself is not. Winnicott often concludes, or begins, his most critical, revisionary papers with a more or less tacit disclaimer, suggesting that his ideas are wholly in agreement with the influential precursors, usually Freud or Klein, of whom he is being critical.

'The Manic Defence' begins as a statement of Winnicott's new-found indebtedness to Klein's ideas which had made real for him, in an unprecedented way, the idea of an inner world. 'In my own particular case,' he writes, 'a widening understanding of Mrs Klein's concept at present named "the manic defence" has coincided with a gradual deepening of my appreciation of inner reality.' Where previously he had contrasted fantasy and reality he has now 'come to compare external reality not so much with fantasy as with an inner reality . . . the change in terminology involves a deepening of belief in inner reality'. For Winnicott, explicitly, a change of language is a change of belief. Melanie Klein has, for him, added to the stock of available reality: now 'it is a part of one's own manic defence to be unable to give full significance to inner reality'.[49] Klein had shown how the child's ongoing, passionate relationship with the parents, felt to be inside him, overlapped with the more obvious relationship to the real external parents. Like the external world, the internal world was only to a very limited extent subject to the infant's control. The infant might, as Winnicott suggests, use fantasy or the external world as bolt-holes from the stress of the inner world. Winnicott distinguishes in his paper two kinds of fantasy. What Klein had called internal reality was represented in 'the fantasy that is personal and organized, and related historically to the physical experiences, excitements, pleasures and pains of infancy'.[50] Then there was the fantasy of daydream, the function of which was to insulate the person from internal reality, from contact with himself and others. For Winnicott, following Klein, it is the pain of desire in its fraught relation with the other, loved person that can turn the external world or the world of omnipotent daydream into a refuge from an inner personal reality. Winnicott gives the accessible example of 'the ordinary extrovert book of adventure' in which

> we often see how the author made a flight to daydreaming in childhood, and then later made use of external reality in this same flight. He is not conscious of the inner depressive anxiety from which he has fled. He has led a life full of incident and adventure, and this may be accurately told. But the impression left on the reader is of a relatively shallow personality, for this very reason, that the author adventurer has had to base his life on the denial of personal internal reality. One turns with relief from such writers to others who can tolerate depressive anxiety and doubt.[51]

What Winnicott eventually called fantasying, and here calls daydreaming, becomes a solution at the cost of personal integrity.[52] But Winnicott implied in 'The Manic Defence', despite his homage to Klein, that she had pathologized normality. Freud had suggested that the ideals civilization imposed on the individual's sexual life were one crucial source of his misery. 'It is one of the obvious social injustices', he wrote, 'that the standard of civilization should demand for everyone the same conduct of sexual life.'[53] The risk of object-relations theory, as formulated by Klein, was that it might create a comparably inappropriate ideal for emotional life. The depressive position, like any formulated standard of the moral life, could merely create the grounds for a new kind of compliance. Psychoanalytic theory could be like an intrusive mother, oppressive in its demands. Klein's views, Winnicott seemed to sense, could constitute another cramping psychoanalytic super-ego, prohibiting common pleasures in the interests of one theory of mental health. He offered the example of the music-hall:

> It should be possible to link the lessening of omnipotent manipulation and of control and of devaluation to normality, and to a degree of manic defence that is employed by all in everyday life. For instance, one is at a music-hall and on to the stage come the dancers, trained to liveliness. One can say that here is the primal scene, here is exhibitionism, here is anal control, here is masochistic submission to discipline, here is a defiance of the super-ego. Sooner or later one adds: here is LIFE. Might it not be that the main point of the performance is a denial of deadness, a defence against depressive 'death inside' ideas, the sexualization being secondary.[54]

In the context of Klein's new-found ascendancy in the British Society it is an appropriately inappropriate example. Entertainment, or the idea of the performing self, is not something one easily associates with Klein's work. Winnicott is saying here that a performance could be valuable *because* it was a denial of deadness. He tries to humanize Klein's harsh rigour by distinguishing between 'normal reassurance through reality' and 'abnormal manic defence'. Winnicott never shared the smug psychoanalytic contempt for the idea of reassurance.

The 'dancers trained to liveliness' – reminiscent of the end of Winnicott's poem, 'To enliven her was my living' –

would return in Winnicott's descriptions of children meeting the depressed mood of their mothers, getting 'caught in with the mother's contra-depressive defences'.[55] Klein's paper had omitted the mother's contribution to the child's organizing of a manic defence. Winnicott was to add to Klein's contribution a manic defence organized to cope with ← the mother's inner reality. His concept of the False Self would cover the child's repertoire of ways of dealing with the mother's intrusive internal reality. In the next decade, from his work with psychotic adults and evacuated children, he would begin to outline his own theory of early emotional development. During the war, of course, it would be increasingly difficult to ignore the pressure of external reality. Winnicott was to become its representative spokesman in the British Society. Margaret Little, one of Winnicott's analysands, recalls that in the first Scientific Meeting of the British Society that she attended, there were 'bombs dropping every few minutes and people ducking as each crash came. In the middle of the discussion someone I later came to know as D. W. stood up and said, "I should like to point out that there is an air-raid going on," and sat down. No notice was taken, and the meeting went on as before!'[56]

My aliveness is in the performance as at Kegs. Liberating from the deadness (miso.) of Nancy.

3 War-time

'Real grievances are displacers of passion.
The imaginary nail a man down for a suf-
ferer, as on a cross; the real spur him up into
an agent.'

John Keats

In December 1939 Winnicott, with two psychiatrists, John
Bowlby and Emmanuel Miller, wrote a letter to the *British
Medical Journal* explaining why 'The evacuation of small
children between the ages of two and five introduces major
psychological problems.' Just as the so-called 'war-neuroses'
had been influential in the development of psychoanalytic
theory, the problems of evacuated children in Britain
changed psychoanalytic thinking about childhood. The
child's premature separation from home could, as the letter
stressed, 'mean far more than the actual experience of
sadness' for the young child; it could in fact 'amount to an
emotional blackout'.[1] The developmental problems of evacuation, for both mothers and children, marked a turning-
point in the work of Bowlby and Winnicott, though not so
obviously in Melanie Klein. Controversy about her work
still raged in the British Society during the war years, and
culminated after the war in the setting up of distinctive
groups within the one British Society. Winnicott, who
would become an important member of the Society after
the war, was to play a role in mediating between these rival
groups. But in 1940 he was appointed Psychiatric Consultant to the Government Evacuation Scheme in the County

of Oxford. It was there that he worked with Clare Britton, the psychiatric social worker for the scheme, who was to become his second wife. From the work he did during the war with psychotic adult patients and homeless children, two groups of people that would become increasingly associated in his mind, he was to clarify his initially tentative differences from Klein and her followers.

Winnicott had emphasized in his work before the war the significance for the child's development of the particular environment, of the mother that was there meeting his need. From Klein's description of the Depressive Position he had come to a more sophisticated awareness of the child's internal world, and the inevitable internal anguish of the infant that was, in psychoanalytic terms, integral to his development. But evacuation was imposed on mothers and children from outside, disrupting the continuity of their relationship (in Winnicott's writing on the subject the plight of fathers is only briefly mentioned). Working with these children and their families, and supervising the hostel-workers' care of the children, put Winnicott in a unique position to assess the relative importance of what he called the 'environmental provision'. Setting up evacuation hostels was, as he wrote, 'an opportunity for experiment in the provision of substitute homes'.[2] And there were comparisons to be made, he found, between the evacuated child in the hostel and the child or adult in the analytic situation. In Winnicott's view the child, like the adult, carried not only his instinctual life but also his early environment inside him and would recreate it in the new situation.[3] So, for example, those children whose placements broke down, he discovered, tended to be those who had never had good-enough care in their original homes. Children with good early experience were 'able to make use of an environment'; they would not feel the pressing need to comply and be used by the environment at the cost of their own needs. In his work with the hostels he could study in a different context what he had observed happening in the psychoanalysis of adults, the child's need 'to build up a belief in his environment'. It was after his work during the war that Winnicott increasingly emphasized something that was central to his sense of what psychoanalysis was about: that for the patient, and this was more true the more disturbed the patient was, the reliability of the setting that the analyst maintains does much of the work of the psychoanalysis. Real development can only come out of, and is the process of finding, belief in the environment. For Winnicott a capacity to be spontaneous can only come out of an early experience of reliability. Only with a backdrop of continuity, one might say, can the patient re-find his own developmental lines. It is worth looking in some detail, then, at this crucial period of Winnicott's work.

Taking for granted that '. . . the younger the child the more danger there is in separating him from his mother', Winnicott had organized the evacuation scheme with two principles in mind. First, 'the fact that children differ from each other widely';[4] and secondly, the issue of what Winnicott called 'the time factor'. There was the simple profound point that, as he wrote, 'time itself is very different according to the age at which it is experienced'.[5] A child's capacity to tolerate waiting, to keep alive the expected mother in his mind as a real and satisfying possibility, was dependent upon both maturity and circumstance. The whole process of leaving home, adapting to the new hostel, and then eventually returning home after a long gap, was potentially fraught with problems that were beyond the child's immature ego to make sense of and therefore allow for. The child needed his personal repertoire of symptoms to deal with the situation. Indeed, for Winnicott it was important it be acknowledged that the child's anti-social behaviour in the new situation was an entirely appropriate response to his loss and deprivation, and was in fact a sign of the child's emotional well-being. The child who could fit in with relative ease to the new environment was, in Winnicott's terms, suffering from a more absolute despair. The absence of symptoms in the evacuated children often revealed deeper problems. The children with symptoms showed a belief in the possibility of a good-enough environment: 'The problem children,' Winnicott wrote, 'because of their nuisance value, had produced a public opinion that would support provision for them which, in fact, catered for their needs.'[6]

In the planning and management of the war-time schemes Winnicott distinguished – and it is a distinction alive in every area of his work – between 'people who are attracted to the task of applying a set scheme' and 'those who are attracted by the task of developing a scheme themselves'.[7] There are those people, Winnicott implies, who recreate what they find out of their own desire, and those who comply by catering excessively to the needs of the environment. From the impinging mother to the indoctrinating analyst, this figure of the rigid, imposing, pre-emptive presence haunts Winnicott's work as a negative ideal, the saboteur of personal development. In a talk written for teachers in 1940, entitled 'Children in the War', Winnicott referred to fascism, for example, as a 'permanent alternative to puberty'.[8] Faced with the management of children deprived of their homes, Winnicott suggested that: 'In all work that concerns the care of human beings it is the worker with originality and a live sense of responsibility that is needed.'[9] Where this was the case residential management itself was a therapy both for the delinquent child and the child made difficult by ordinary home-sickness. In his later work on delinquency Winnicott would write that psychotherapy with this particular group of people was only possible, was in fact subsidized, by placement of the child in a setting in which he could rely on firm but sympathetic management. The early precursor of this kind of management, in Winnicott's terms, was the mother's holding of her child in a way that made him feel safe without his having to submit to her constraint. In the hostels, Winnicott wrote in 'The Problem of Homeless Children', at best 'the children get consistent and continuous management ... it is the permanent nature of the home that makes it valuable even more than the fact that the work is done intelligently.'[10]

Winnicott explained the role of the various members of staff in the hostel in a way that makes sense of his oddly bureaucratic term 'management', and offered by implication his notions of good parenting. The psychiatric social worker, 'as far as the children are concerned is to give them a sense of continuity throughout the changes to which they are subjected'. She was the link with the child's parents and so was 'able in some degree to gather together the separate threads of the child's life and to give him the opportunity of preserving something important to him from each stage of his experience'.[11] Winnicott was always attentive to the young child's need for an adult to hold together the threads of his experience. The mother, for example, can keep the story of the child's experience alive and viable by putting it together and telling it back when the child needs to know.

They had found that the choice of warden for the hostels was not a question of training, or education, or interests. It was, in fact, 'impossible to generalize about the type of person who makes a good warden', though the qualities they described him as needing represent what would become familiar as a maternal ego-ideal in Winnicott's work. A warden must have, they wrote:

> the ability to assimilate experience, and to deal in a genuine, spontaneous way with the events and relationships of life. This is of the utmost importance, for only

those who are confident enough to be themselves and
to act in a natural way can act consistently day in and
day out . . . We must point out, however, that there will
be times when the warden will have to 'act naturally'
in the sense that an actor acts naturally.[12]

One of Winnicott's insistent preoccupations was with the
description of a character defined both by certain essential
qualities – he or she tends to be genuine, personal, spontaneous, natural, confident, and open to experience – with the
perhaps related but paradoxical ability to 'act' these same
qualities. In the example here the warden – like the mother
and the analyst – has to be able to 'act' naturally as part of
his adaptation to the children who are 'too ill or too anxious
to be able to allow for the warden's own personal difficulties
as well as their own'.[13] 'Acting' in this context is being able
willingly, and not compulsively, to adapt for the sake of the
child's developmental needs; just as the analyst might, at
times, fit in with the patient.

The consistency of the residential setting was bound up
with Winnicott's conception of what he calls in this paper
the True Nature of Home. In this good-enough environment
the child can only believe in and trust his parents if they
afford him opportunity to test their goodness. And this
involves allowing for what Winnicott calls elsewhere
'almost . . . the child's most sacred attribute: doubts about
self'.[14] The child must, he writes, 'test over and over again
their ability to remain good parents in spite of anything he
may do to hurt or annoy them. By means of this testing he
gradually convinces himself, if the parents do in fact stand
the strain.'[15] The parents, that is to say, are consistently
resilient, and not rejecting of the child. Winnicott is clear
that only the child's real parents are likely to be able to give
him so much. But Winnicott uses this description of the
real home as a model for what he calls the three phases of

the child's usual response to being placed in the hostel. Winnicott was increasingly interested in the sequence of developmental processes in the child's life. These three phases are the first of a series we will find in Winnicott's work. The three phases Winnicott describes here are, in abbreviated form, as follows:

1. 'For the first short phase the child is extraordinarily normal . . . he has new hope, he scarcely sees people as they are, and the staff and the other children have not yet had any reason to begin to disillusion him . . . It is a dangerous stage because what he sees and responds to in the warden and his staff is his ideal of what a good father and mother would be like.'

2. At this stage there is for the child 'the breaking down of his ideal. He sets about this first by testing the building and the people physically. He wants to know what damage he can do, and how much he can do with impunity. Then if he finds that he can be physically managed, that is, that the place and the people in it have nothing to fear from him physically, he starts to test by subtlety, putting one member of the staff against another . . . trying to make people give each other away, and doing all he can to get favoured himself.'

3. And finally, 'If the hostel withstands these tests the child enters the third phase, settles down with a sigh of relief, and joins in the life of the group as an ordinary member.'[16]

It is worth noting in Winnicott's account that the child needs to test the environment: the child, in Winnicott's view, is in search of reality, not attempting to escape from it. He needs to know that the environment can withstand him. Winnicott uses the sequence he has described to identify a group of children he will call 'anti-social'. Because of an early deprivation, the anti-social child 'will be

68

specially active in testing his environment'. 'Even when the environment stands up to the test,' he writes, 'anti-social children cannot believe this fact for more than a short length of time.'[17] But he emphasizes that their persistence is a sign of hope, of a belief in finding the holding environment they require. 'The anti-social tendency', Winnicott writes, 'is a reaction to *deprivation*, not a result of privation; [it] . . . belongs to the stage of relative (not absolute) dependence.'[18] It implies, in other words, that the anti-social child is trying to re-find something good that he once had.

Returning home was also, potentially, a new opportunity for the child, provided, Winnicott said in a radio talk to parents, 'the child can take time to get to feel that what *is* real is real. This does take time, and you must allow for a slow dawning of confidence.'[19] The process by which the child, and then the adult, finds what is real to him was to be at the centre of the developmental theory Winnicott would formulate after the war. And we will see Winnicott observe in close detail the ordinary infant's 'slow dawning of confidence' in relation to his own desire and the consequent need for an environment that allows for the infant's pauses and hesitations and regressions as part of the process. But Winnicott tried to convey, from the child's point of view, what returning home might be like after a long separation. He makes the paradoxical point that the child's growing confidence will be reflected in his increasing willingness to be difficult. 'He may very likely try out a little thieving,' Winnicott says, 'testing how true it is that you are really his mother, and so in a sense what is yours is his.'[20] Like the infant, the returning child needs to believe again in a mother upon whom he can make absolute claims; what might be called, given Winnicott's suggestive phrasing, his infantile marital rights. But it is the parent's withstanding of the child's aggressive non-compliance – not simply what Klein would call his 'innate sadism' – that

69

brings Winnicott to a striking and stark formulation that he can only offer as a question: 'Shall I say that, for a child to be brought up so that he can discover the deepest part of his nature, someone has to be defied, and even at times hated, without there being a danger of a complete break in the relationship?'[21] Clearly not all parents are concerned about bringing up their children to be able to discover what Winnicott considers to be 'the deepest parts of their nature'. But what Winnicott proposes here is the developmental necessity of an acknowledged and perhaps innate non-compliance in the child that is bound up with aggression, but the aggression that is integral to the drive for personal development. It was to be the relationship between the infant's primitive, ruthless love – the greed that Winnicott called 'mouth love' – and the infant's potential for compliance that Winnicott was to put at the centre of his distinctive developmental theory.

II

In a paper written in 1940 called 'Discussion of War Aims',[22] Winnicott links 'the importance of greed in human affairs', the greed that is 'love in a primitive form', with issues about personal freedom now prompted by the rise of fascism in Europe. Our attitude to instinctual life, he suggests, of which greed is the most primitive form, contains an obvious contradiction. We value one idea of freedom that is bound up with the freedom for instinctual expression and yet we are also afraid, so much so that we 'tend at times to be drawn towards being controlled'. He proposes, with the boldness that characterized early 'applied' psychoanalysis, that the fascist state is a false solution for the individual to the 'fear of chaos and uncontrol' that the earliest instinctual life brings with it. This fear generates either 'the compulsion to attain power' or the need to be controlled. 'Both inhibition and licence', Winnicott writes, 'are easy, and both may be cheaply bought by giving over responsibility to an idealized leader or to a principle; but the result is poverty of personality.'[23] The question evolving out of Winnicott's work was: how does a person grow from a state of primitive greed and absolute dependence on the mother to relative autonomy in which he can acknowledge the existence of other people without too much loss of spontaneity and desire – without the false solution of a rigid conviction or a strong leader? It was the point at which psychoanalytic ideas about development joined up with the then threatened idea of democracy. In a paper written in 1950 Winnicott would suggest that there was a precarious but 'innate democratic tendency'[24] in the developing individual.

In the 'Discussion of War Aims' Winnicott made a distinction that would run through his later work and that revealed his distrust of, or dismay about, the nature of instinctual life. 'There can be', he wrote, 'a wide discrepancy between what we like when we are excited and what we like interim.' There is a difference between the quiescent self and the excited self. Winnicott says in this paper that instinctual life is an 'interference with the exercise and enjoyment of freedom'; that 'there is but little bodily gratification, and none that is acute, to be got out of freedom'.[25] Excitement tends to turn up in object-relations theory as a defence against something reputedly more valuable. It was in fact to the uses of excitement that object-relations theorists turned their attention. The implication of Winnicott's remarks in this early paper is that freedom is freedom from bodily excitement. As though in states of desire the self was, as it were, complying with the tyranny of the body. It was the self relatively uncomplicated by desire – the child absorbed in play, the experience of friendship, the 'ego-orgasm' – that Winnicott described as 'a highly satisfactory experience such as may be obtained at a concert or at the theatre';[26] these kinds of experience, and

71

ruth less
ness
?

not what he called 'id-relationships', would tend to constitute his version of the good life. It was, however, the revelations of appetite, the study of greed that was at the same time the study of the first relationship, that would enable Winnicott to formulate his developmental theory.

'Simply following the lead given by careful history-taking in innumerable cases,' Winnicott had realized, as he writes in 'Appetite and Emotional Disorder', 'the full importance of eating'. 'If I wish to describe a little child,' he adds, 'I must show you something of his oral interests.'[27] Where Freud had found that all neurotics suffered from some disturbance in their sexual life, Winnicott pointed out that, faced with an ill child or even a relatively normal child, it was 'quite rare to get a history . . . that does not reveal feeding symptoms'. The infant's attitude to food, his use of appetite, would inevitably be a precursor of later relationships — relationships with other people, but also with his own desire. In this relatively early paper, written in 1936, Winnicott gave the first detailed description of a process he would later formalize in one of his most important papers, 'The Observation of Infants in a Set Situation' (1941).[28] The later, more organized statement was given to the British Psychoanalytical Society; it is instructive in this particular case to look at the account he was freer to give in the earlier paper to the Medical Section of the British Psychological Society.

From his work in his hospital out-patient clinic he wants to 'convey an impression of the morning's pageant'. He has noticed that the way a child finds and uses the spatulas he puts on his desk helps him to understand the child's development — that 'deviations from this mean of behaviour indicate deviations from normal emotional development'. What Winnicott describes is striking in two ways. First, it is extremely simple and requires minimal active intervention by the doctor; and secondly, it is a performance in which the child's and the therapist's use of the audience as environment is integral to the event. ('Everyone is now in hilarious mood,' Winnicott remarks towards the end of one case description, 'the clinic is going very well.') This is the account of the process in which the audience of the paper, the environment in which it was received, made possible a less inhibited and more concise picture than the official statement to the British Society:

... I want to give an account of what a baby does as he sits on his mother's lap with the corner of the table between them and me.

A child of one year behaves in the following way. He sees the spatula and soon puts his hand to it, but he probably withdraws interest once or twice, before actually taking it, all the while looking at my face and at his mother's to gauge our attitudes. Sooner or later he takes it and mouths it. He now enjoys possession of it and at the same time he kicks and shows eager bodily activity. He is not yet ready to have it taken away from him. Soon he drops the spatula on the floor; first this may seem like a chance happening, but as it is restored to him he eventually repeats the mistake, and at last he throws it down and obviously intends that it shall drop. He looks at it, and often the noise of its contact with the floor becomes a new source of joy for him. He will like to throw it down repeatedly if I give him the chance. He now wants to get down to be with it on the floor ... What he does with the spatula (or with anything else) between the taking and the dropping is a film-strip of the little bit of his inner world that is related to me and his mother at that time, and from this can be guessed a good deal about his inner world experiences at other times and in relation to other people and things.[29]

Winnicott makes it clear that the mothers and children in the adjoining room participate; 'the mood of the whole room is determined', he writes, 'by the baby's mood. A mother over the way says: "He's the village blacksmith,"' and the baby she is referring to, Winnicott says, 'is pleased at such success and adds to his play an element of showing off'. Winnicott notes how a more inhibited, unhappy child 'creates an abnormal environment for himself' by using the spatula in a way that for the audience 'means something to do with masturbation'. Winnicott notices that the other parents distract their children from the sight of him so that 'the little boy finds himself in company in which no one gives him the reassurance he so desperately needs'.[30] As with the evacuated children in the hostel, Winnicott is attentive to the kind of environment the child creates for himself, how he discovers and uses what he finds, as the essential indicator of emotional development.

Winnicott pays close attention to the three stages of the process, as the child moves from the first 'timid approach' to a degree of confidence, 'mouthing . . . and live play', through to the child finishing with the spatula. How the child involves, by invitation and refusal, the witnesses; the degree and kind of reassurance the child seeks from the environment; how free the child is in his use of the spatula; all these are telling details. And they can be easily translated, as Winnicott implies, to the adult or child patient's use of the analyst and his interpretations. What Winnicott calls 'the first stage of timid approach', and later in the same paper refers to as the 'period of suspicion', he calls in 'The Observation of Infants' 'the period of hesitation'. His successive redescription of this first moment reflects its significance for Winnicott. What may look, from a more orthodox psychoanalytic point of view, like a defensive resistance in the patient in analysis, may in fact be a period of hesitation, a slow coming to realization, that needs to be allowed for, given time, and not interpreted as evasive. Resistance can reflect the untimeliness, and therefore the irrelevance, of the analyst's interpretation. For Winnicott the patient is not intrinsically unacceptable to himself, but he can only come to himself in his own time. As Winnicott remarks, he cannot force the spatula into the child's mouth.

In his more official statement to the British Society, Winnicott fills in the three stages of the process in more detail. He underplays the element of performance and stresses in what he calls this 'given situation which is easily staged' how important it is for the infant that the 'full course of an experience is allowed'.[31] In a section entitled 'Whole Experiences' he uses the example of the spatula game to add something to the picture he was always building up of a good environment:

> In the intuitive management of an infant a mother naturally allows the full course of the various experiences, keeping this up until the infant is old enough to understand her point of view. She hates to break into such experiences as feeding or sleeping or defecating. In my observations I artificially give the baby the right to complete an experience which is of particular value to him as an object lesson.[32]

Psychoanalytic treatment was, in a comparable way for Winnicott, the allowance of time, 'the analyst lets the patient set the pace'. In fact the infant's use of the spatula provides a clarifying analogy for the analytic process. Despite the 'multitude of details' in the analysis it could nevertheless, he suggests, 'be thought of in the same terms as those in which one can think of the relatively simple set situation which I have described. Each interpretation is a glittering object which excites the patient's greed.'[33] Winnicott implies here that it is not the interpretation in itself that matters but the patient's use of the interpretation.

What he makes of what he's given – the 'glittering object' – is more significant than the given thing.

But the child's capacity to use objects, like the adult's capacity to use analysis, depended upon the successful negotiation of the very earliest stages of development. Only Melanie Klein had provided a psychoanalytic account of the infant, as opposed to the child. Winnicott now felt in a position to challenge this with a developmental theory of his own.

III

Winnicott's paper of 1945, 'Primitive Emotional Development',[34] is a watershed in his work. It gathers together twenty years of clinical experience as a psychoanalyst and paediatrician, and provides a ground-plan for all his later speculation. As the most cursory reading of Klein's rival paper, 'Notes on Some Schizoid Mechanisms',[35] published the following year, will reveal, it is distinctive in its relative disregard for the language of Freudian and Kleinian metapsychology. Winnicott's terms – integration, personalization, realization, illusion, disillusionment, ruthlessness – are accessible because they are familiar from other contexts. Unlike Klein he is explicit that his position is based on ignorance, that 'there is a great deal that is not known or properly understood' about the earliest developmental stages.

Klein and her followers had found, from the psychoanalysis of psychotic adult patients, what they claimed was a replication of the earliest stages of infancy. From Klein's point of view, at the very earliest stages of development the infant could be described as psychotic. Winnicott, who had been primarily interested in infants and children, had decided he needed therefore to study psychosis in adults.

His paper, he says, came out of the work he did with twelve psychotic adult patients during the war. 'I hardly noticed the blitz,' he writes, 'being all the time engaged in the analysis of psychotic patients who are notoriously and maddeningly oblivious of bombs, earthquakes and floods.'[36] This obliviousness to the external world was integral, of course, to Winnicott's enquiry, into the role of the environment in the most severe states of psychopathology. Was what Klein had described as psychosis in adults a consequence of early environmental privation rather than of a putative innate tendency observable in the ordinary infant? Winnicott had found that psychosis in adults was the result of early maternal failure.

Winnicott begins his paper by pointing out that there had been more or less consensual agreement among psychoanalysts that 'at five to six months a change occurs in infants which makes it more easy than before for us to refer to their emotional development in the terms that apply to human beings generally'.[37] Though they had formulated it in quite different terms, this was the period at which for Klein, Anna Freud and Bowlby, the infant became able to acknowledge the distinct existence of the mother as a separate person. 'At this stage', Winnicott writes, 'a baby becomes able in his play to show that he can understand that he has an inside, and that things come from outside.'[38] It is imagined that the infant has begun to evolve fantasies about boundaries, and these fantasies revolve around the mother, the first bit of the outside world that enters the orbit of his awareness. 'The corollary of this', Winnicott writes, 'is that now the infant assumes that his mother also has an inside, one which may be rich or poor, good or bad, ordered or muddled. He is therefore starting to be concerned with the mother and her sanity and moods.'[39] This new capacity to be preoccupied by another person imagined as comparable to oneself is a considerable achievement. For Winnicott the six-month stage is a relatively sophisticated one, as it was for Klein, in terms of emotional development. But his thesis in this paper is that the earlier stage, 'before the infant knows himself (and therefore others) as the whole person that he is (and that they are) is vitally important; indeed that here are the clues to the psychopathology of psychosis'.[40] And this earlier stage, of course, is the one in which it can be said that the mother can know her infant but the infant cannot know his mother: a period, from Winnicott's point of view, of ultimate maternal responsibility.

Klein was to propose, as an account of the infant's earliest state of mind, what she called the paranoid-schizoid position. Through the mechanisms that constituted this stage – splitting and idealization – the infant was supposed to manage his ambivalence to maintain his nurture. The infant's initial developmental project was to deal with the psychic pain consequent upon his innate sadism. In Winnicott's quite different model the infant's project was, through sufficient maternal care, to inhabit his body. And the body was not constituted for Winnicott, as it was for Klein, by instinctual life; it was not the site of a battle between the Life instincts and the Death instincts. Winnicott put at the centre of his developmental model not a mythic conflict between incompatible forces but 'the localization of self in one's body'.[41] In the work of Freud and Klein it was difficult to find a use for the idea of a Self; the essential terms were the idea of the unconscious and the instincts, and the unconscious seemed by definition to preclude the validity of any unitary self. For Winnicott there was the body at the root of development out of which a 'psycho-somatic partnership' evolved. The self was first and foremost a body self and the 'psyche' of the partnership 'means the imaginative elaboration of somatic parts, feelings and functions, that is, of physical aliveness'.[42] 'The psyche and the soma', he wrote, 'have to come to terms with each other,'[43] and this coming to terms, this finding of a shared language, was the developmental process. The 'establishment of a firm relationship'[44] between psyche and soma was not, for Winnicott, an exclusively conflictual process. With good-enough maternal care at the earliest stages the building up of the self was a process of natural coordination. And this process of coordination was itself constituted by three processes that 'start very early: (1) integration, (2) personalization, and, (3) following these, the appreciation of time and space and other properties of reality – in short, realization'.[45]

At the very beginning, Winnicott suggests, the infant is in a condition of 'primary unintegration', by which he means unconnected feeling states and without even a rudimentary ego. In a Winnicottian baby's life there are long periods when he is just a bundle of disparate feelings and impressions and he doesn't, as an adult would say, mind that this is the case provided, Winnicott writes, 'from time to time he comes together and feels something'. He has, every so often, what can be thought of as unifying experiences that come from without and from within. This natural 'tendency to integrate' is made possible by the mother's care in which the infant is 'kept warm, handled and bathed and rocked and named', and also by 'acute instinctual experiences which tend to gather the personality together from within'. 'Rest for the infant', he writes, 'means a return to an unintegrated state'[46] (it is important to remember here that the infant at rest was of little interest to Klein). These two parallel orders of event – ordinary care and instinctual experience – repeated over time, gather together the 'many bits' of the baby into a person capable of being occasionally 'one whole being'. With 'one person (the mother) to gather his bits together', the infant has available the possibility of being both 'all over the place' and someone

79

in particular whom we would at a later stage describe as having their feet on the ground. 'It is instinctual experience and the repeated quiet experiences of body care', Winnicott writes, 'that gradually build up what may be called satisfactory personalization.'[47] There is a dawning sense of being a specific person whose particularity is rooted in his body and which will be elaborated into the sentiment of being who one happens to be. And this involves, at a very early stage, being able, with increasing competence, to orientate oneself in time and space. Winnicott is careful to distinguish unintegration from the psychopathological state of disintegration. Unintegration means being able to entrust oneself to an environment in which one can safely and easily be in bits and pieces without the feeling of falling apart. Disintegration signifies a failure of the holding environment and is, as Winnicott writes in a later paper,

> a sophisticated *defence*, a defence that is an active production of chaos in defence against unintegration in the absence of maternal ego-support, that is, against the unthinkable or archaic anxiety that results from failure of holding in the stage of absolute dependence. The chaos of disintegration may be as 'bad' as the unreliability of the environment, but it has the advantage of being produced by the baby and therefore of being non-environmental. It is within the reach of the baby's omnipotence.[48]

Unintegration is a resource, disintegration is a terror. Winnicott insists that a capacity for states of primary unintegration brought forward into later life is a developmental necessity. He refers to 'much sanity that has a symptomatic quality being charged with fear or denial of madness, fear or denial of the innate capacity of every human being to become unintegrated, depersonalized, and to feel that the world is unreal'.[49] And to this Winnicott adds a rightly famous footnote: 'Through artistic expression we can hope to keep in touch with our primitive selves whence the most intense feelings and even fearfully acute sensations derive, and we are poor indeed if we are only sane.' Winnicott equates the intensity of feeling of these primitive selves with a madness that he conceives of as nourishing. In our more purposive states of mind we are held together; the risk, Winnicott implies, is that we will impose a coherence on ourselves that can divorce us from our more 'primitive selves'.

So for Winnicott the healthy integration made possible by a holding environment is always reversible; states of unintegration can be tolerated and enjoyed. But if integration is 'incomplete or partial' the unintegrated parts of the infant become, in Winnicott's view, dissociated. In dissociation the unintegrated parts of the self lose touch with the developmental process that links them. It is as though they are adrift somewhere unknown though still in the orbit of the self, so an adult patient, for example, may be occasionally aware of what feels like an unknowable deficit in himself, and yet be unable to elaborate a representation of it. Winnicott gives as a more ordinary example the fact that for a child there is not necessarily a connection in his mind between himself asleep and himself awake. They are at first dissociated states and the dissociation only begins to break down, he writes, when dreams are remembered and 'conveyed' to another person. 'Children depend', he writes, 'very much on adults for getting to know their dreams . . . It is a valuable experience whenever a dream is both dreamed and remembered, precisely because of the breakdown of dissociation this represents.'[50] This, of course, would be the ordinary precursor of dream-interpretation in analysis in which it is the patient's 'conveying' of the dream that it is the function of the analyst's interpretation to acknowledge. Psychoanalysis becomes, on the basis of Winnicott's developmental model, the connecting of dissociated parts of the self and not modifying the repression of instincts.

But the early dissociation in the personality that preoccupies Winnicott is that between 'the quiet and the excited states' of the infant. He is not at first aware that when he is enjoying being bathed or stroked or warm he is the same person who can be 'screaming for immediate satisfaction, possessed by an urge to get at and destroy something unless satisfied by milk'.[51] It is as though he imagines that the two parts of himself correspond to two different mothers. 'He does not know at first', Winnicott writes, 'that the mother he is building up through his quiet experiences is the same as the power behind the breasts that he has in his mind to destroy.'[52] As we shall see in the next chapter, this, for Winnicott, is the fundamental dissociation in the personality, and it is dissociation – not repression, or splitting, both of which imply an ego to do the work – that for Winnicott precludes further development. Only 'after integration', he writes in a later paper, 'the infant begins to have a self'.[53] And integration means literally the combining of parts.

If integration can be assumed then the next step for the infant is what Winnicott calls 'another enormous subject, the primary relation to external reality', a relation he regards as 'never finally made and settled'. It is integral to Winnicott's approach that developmental stages do not progressively dispense with each other but are included in a personal repertoire. Maturity is then the flexible toleration of, and potential access to, a full and ever-increasing repertoire throughout life. So-called developmental achievements are only achievements for Winnicott if they are reversible. So a relation with external reality is dependent upon a capacity to relinquish this relation in a return to states of primary unintegration in which one can be, for example, 'miles away', or simply preoccupied.

Winnicott suggests that the infant's preliminary contact

with external reality is made possible by what he calls 'moments of illusion'. We usually think of an illusion as something deceptive, or as something we may believe in to protect ourselves from a more unacceptable reality. In Winnicott's idiosyncratic use of the word it is by way of illusion, and indeed only through illusion, that the infant can get to reality. Winnicott imagines that when the infant is hungry he fantasizes a satisfying breast, at which point the real breast is made available by the mother. In this moment of illusion it is as though, from the infant's point of view, he has created the mother he eats. 'At the start,' Winnicott writes, 'simple contact with external or shared reality has to be made by the infant's hallucinating and the world's presenting, with moments of illusion for the infant in which the two are taken by him to be identical, which they never in fact are.'[54] By 'hallucinating', here Winnicott means that the infant imaginatively creates the breast out of his desire for it. Through the mother's empathic identification with the desire of her infant he can believe, when he is hungry, that he has made what he has, in fact, found. But this essential moment of illusion requires the overlap of two desires:

> . . . the baby has instinctual urges and predatory ideas. The mother has a breast and the power to produce milk, and the idea that she would like to be attacked by a hungry baby. These two phenomena do not come into relation with each other till the mother and child *live an experience together*. I think of the process as if two lines came from opposite directions, liable to come near each other. If they overlap there is a moment of *illusion* – a bit of experience which the infant can take as *either* his hallucination *or* a thing belonging to external reality.[55]

To create the moment of illusion requires two participants that from the infant's point of view look like only one; the mother enters the scene as a desiring subject, desiring, that is to say, to be eaten, and by doing so she realizes the infant's fantasy. By virtue of her 'sensitive adaptation', fantasy, in its original form, is the infant's route to reality, his medium of contact. 'Fantasy', Winnicott writes, 'is more primary than reality, and the enrichment of fantasy with the world's riches depends on the experience of illusion.'[56] The infant can only tolerate, at first, being nourished by an object he appears to possess and control, so the mother fits in with his desire. Only this repeated experience gives him confidence in his desire as a source of possibility. Only if the object has been known to be there when desired can it gradually be waited for and eventually longed for; only then does the child's inner world find an incentive for contact with the external world. Because his desire has been met and satisfied he has had the primitive experience of a match between inner and outer. The Kleinian infant, we remember, by virtue of his desire, was a misfit. So development for Winnicott begins with a magical act: the infant's purely imaginative process of conjuring up a mother he needs. At the very beginning fantasy is not a substitute for reality but the first method of finding it.

It is what Winnicott refers to as the 'mother's job' at the beginning 'to protect her infant from complications that cannot yet be understood by the infant, and to go on steadily providing the simplified bit of the world which the infant, through her, comes to know'.[57] The mother, in a sense, sustains the infant's capacity for illusion, his capacity for exchange with the external world, by keeping the world she presents to him simple; she doesn't make demands upon him or subject him to experiences that are beyond his tolerance or comprehension. Because of the infant's need for simple and reliable continuity of care, Winnicott stresses that in his view the infant needs one caretaker, preferably his own mother, whose particular adaptation to his need can become familiar. Then the infant's fantasy can be 'enriched by actual details of sight, smell, feel, and next time this material is used in the hallucination. In this way [the infant] starts to build up a capacity to conjure up what is actually available.' In Freud, reality is that which frustrates the individual; in Winnicott's account, at the very beginning at least, reality is both potentially enriching and also reassuring in the way it sets limits to fantasy. It is not something inexorable to which a person must comply but can be something a person can use for satisfaction. Referring to Freud (and not, of course, only to Freud), Winnicott writes,

> We often hear of the very real frustrations imposed by external reality, but less often hear of the relief and satisfaction it affords. Real milk is satisfying as compared with imaginary milk, but this is not the point. The point is that in fantasy things work by magic: there are no brakes on fantasy, and love and hate cause alarming effects. External reality has brakes on it, and can be studied and known, and, in fact, fantasy is only tolerable at full blast when objective reality is appreciated well. The subjective has tremendous value but is so alarming and magical that it cannot be enjoyed except as a parallel to the objective.[58]

Insofar as external reality demanded submission or compliance it was, Winnicott wrote, the 'arch-enemy of spontaneity, creativity and the sense of Real'.[59] The Reality Principle as 'the fact of the existence of the world whether the baby creates it or not' could only be experienced, he wrote, as 'an insult'.[60] But if the mother has provided her infant with the opportunity for illusion, and dosed his experience of reality – that which eludes his control – reality has the potential to be both nourishing and comforting. It represents for the growing child a promising invitation.

What is often referred to by Winnicott's admirers and critics alike – the apparently reassuring account he gives of early infancy – must be seen in part as, perhaps, a typically English attempt to restore a balance. It is a position that is reactive to Klein's account of the infant as psychotic. Against Klein, Winnicott suggests that the infant, with a sufficiently responsive and caring mother, is not innately unacceptable or terrifying to himself. 'Ordinary babies', he stresses, 'are not mad.'[61] Infantile desire is not in and of itself intolerable, but the infant's attitude, so to speak, to his own desire is constituted by the mother's reception of it. Winnicott does not talk in his paper on primitive emotional development of innate sadism or a paranoid-schizoid position; indeed, what Klein called the paranoid-schizoid position could in Winnicott's terms be the description of an infant simply kept waiting too long by an inattentive mother. Instead of innate sadism Winnicott 'postulates an early ruthless object relationship' which is part of the ordinary infant's benign exploitation of the mother. 'The normal child', he writes, 'enjoys a ruthless relation to his mother, mostly showing in play, and he needs his mother because only she can be expected to tolerate his ruthless relation to her even in play, because this really hurts her and wears her out.'[62]

As we shall see, it takes Winnicott a long time to come to a relatively clear statement about the ruthlessness of the primitive love impulse. One of his most significant contributions to psychoanalytic theory, it was, by the same token, a most troubling idea to him that concern for the object could be a developmental inhibition. In this early statement his equivocation is itself revealing. On the one hand he writes, with defensive firmness, 'certainly no one can be ruthless after the concern stage except in a dissociated state';[63] and then in the following sentence he says that these ruthless dissociation states are 'common in early childhood, and emerge in certain types of delinquency, and madness, and must be available in health'. Winnicott's work after the war can be seen as a growing tolerance, through the process of theoretical elaboration, of the idea of the ruthless early relationship to the mother as integral to development. In the important papers written in the late 1940s he tries to describe the vital connection between the infant's primitive ruthlessness and the continuity of care on which his development depends. It is the mother's capacity to adapt to her infant, which includes surviving his ruthlessness, that facilitates or sabotages the connection. Winnicott's work with psychotic adult patients, like his work with evacuated children, had reinforced his sense that it was the environmental provision and not exclusively the human constitution, as constructed in psychoanalysis, that made for psychopathology.

IV

For Winnicott the mother–infant relationship was becoming the primary model for the psychoanalytic situation; it was, quite literally, the source of analogy in his work. His new ideas about early development and psychosis as an 'environmental deprivation disease' necessarily involved modifications of the classical psychoanalytic technique Freud had invented for the analysis of neurotics. If, as Winnicott now believed, the mother herself played such a decisive role in the infant's development, then when the earliest relationships were recreated in the analytic setting new demands would be made on the analyst. What the patient transferred on to the analyst from his past, and how the analyst was to respond, were becoming pressing ques-

87

tions in the British Society. The Klein group insisted that the analysis of psychotic patients required no essential modification of classical technique. Winnicott made explicit his own sense of these issues in what was, by psychoanalytic standards, a radically self-revealing paper, entitled 'Hate in the Countertransference' (1947).[64] In the analysis of psychotics, he wrote, 'quite a different type and degree of strain is taken by the analyst', and it was to an understanding of this strain that Winnicott turned his attention.

The analyst of a psychotic adult patient must, Winnicott writes, 'be prepared to bear a strain without expecting the patient to know anything about what he is doing, perhaps over a long period of time. To do this he must be easily aware of his own fear and hate. *He is in the position of the mother of an infant unborn or newly born.*'[65] (My italics.)

In this new model of the analytic setting, devised for the psychotic patient, the setting is not symbolic of the mother's care as it would be with a neurotic patient, it *is* the mother's care. It cannot represent something that never existed. The earliest experiences of the psychotic patient – the mothering that should have facilitated the processes of integration, personalization and realization – 'have been so deficient or distorted that the analyst has to be the first in the patient's life to supply certain environmental essentials'.[66] The analytic setting provides the medium for growth that was absent for the patient at the very beginning. The implicit analogy, as usual with Winnicott, is with simpler forms of organic life; the belated provision of the right soil for the plant (and the analogy, of course, suggests the risk that the analyst will begin to identify himself with a fantasy of the all-powerful mother). Freud had invented the psychoanalytic method for neurotic patients which was characterized by the analyst's interpretation of the patient's repressed unconscious. Winnicott was describing a setting that restored an environment – restored it for the first time, so to speak – in which development could start up again. A regression was supposed to occur in which verbal interpretation was secondary to care in a broader, maternal sense; and at certain stages in the treatment, as one would find as the mother of an infant or small child, 'the analyst's hate is actually sought by the patient'. Winnicott offers the analogy of a child from a broken home to reach the surprising conclusion that is the main point of his paper:

> It is notoriously inadequate to take such a child into one's home and love him. What happens is that after a while a child so adopted gains hope, and then he starts to test out the environment he has found, and to seek proof of his guardian's ability to hate objectively. It seems that he can believe in being loved only after reaching being hated.[67]

If he is not hated, if what is unacceptable about him is not acknowledged, then his love and loveableness will not feel fully real to him. What Winnicott calls 'hating appropriately', that is carried over into the psychoanalytic treatment of psychotic adults, is a function of the real relationship. Where Klein had built her theory around the infant's destructiveness towards the mother, Winnicott proposed the opposite alternative: 'I suggest that the mother hates the baby before the baby hates the mother, and before the baby knows the mother hates him.'[68] In Winnicott's terms the notion of 'hate' implies a relatively late stage of development which includes a relationship with a whole other person and an intention to hurt. At the very beginning for Winnicott there is not 'hate' but primitive love, and this ruthless demand must evoke the hatred of the mother; it is the turning of this hatred against herself and not against the infant that Winnicott regards as the source of so-called female masochism. He lists eighteen strong reasons why the mother ordinarily hates her infant and they are all the consequence of his ruthless use of her in the service of his own development. Optimally, just like the analyst of the psychotic patient, she must not retaliate beyond the infant's capacity to make sense of her feelings. From the infant's point of view he is simply loving the mother; from the mother's point of view it can feel like a ruthless assault in which the infant cannot, and must not be made to, empathize or identify with the mother. As there must be in the analysis of psychotics 'avoidance of therapy that is adapted to the needs of the therapist rather than to the needs of the patient',[69] so, in Winnicott's parallel model of mothering, it is, at the very beginning, an act of supreme sacrifice and self-control. The mother, in this excessively demanding account, must allow herself to be used in the service of the developmental process. She is, as it were, continuously giving birth to her infant.

In a complementary paper written the following year, 'Reparation in Respect of Mother's Organized Defence against Depression',[70] Winnicott writes about the infant or child with a depressed mother. His theoretical work now had a distinctive preoccupation with the impact of the mother's feelings on the infant, and the distortions of development that were a consequence of the child's having to manage the mother's moods. Though her hatred, presented in tolerable doses, was integral to the child's development, her depression could be a demand that sabotaged it. And Winnicott used these ideas, more boldly than before, as a way of understanding Klein's position in the British Society. Having described in detail the effect of the depressed mother on the child, he concludes his paper with a plea that, 'each individual member of our Society must achieve his *own* growth at his *own* pace.'[71] The implication is that Klein's followers had been suffering from her depression at the cost of their own individual potential. Children with depressed mothers, Winnicott writes, 'have a task which can never be accomplished. Their task is first to deal with mother's mood.'[72] 'Has due recognition been given', Winnicott asks pointedly, 'to the need for everything to be discovered afresh by every individual analyst?'[73] It was a position reactive to a Society which had, in Winnicott's view, equated development within a tradition with an uncritical compliance to the tradition. Winnicott was beginning to cure himself of Klein.

Where Klein had put the infant's capacity for depression at the centre of her work, Winnicott began to take seriously the effect of the mother's depression on the infant. Psychopathology, in his view, referred to the ways in which the infant or child complied with demands from the environment that were extrinsic to his real development; and one of the functions of this compliance was to protect a possibility for future growth in a more nurturing environment. The normal infant, by natural right, Winnicott believed, used his mother unconditionally for his own growth. But if the mother was depressed and unable to adapt and respond to her infant, the process was reversed and the mother used the child to sustain something in herself. After all, in the mother–infant couple there was always an overlap of two sets of developmental needs, it was not only the infant who was developing. Just as Klein had paid little attention to the person of the mother and saw psychoanalysis, along classical lines, as the interpretation of the transference, so, by the same token, the person of the analyst was relatively anonymous in her account of the process. But Winnicott's enquiries into the earliest mother–infant relationship brought up difficult issues about the reciprocities in the analytic treatment that the classical model evolved by Freud and espoused by Klein had managed to avoid. What was the analyst's desire *vis à vis* the patient, what was the analyst using the patient for, how did the patient figure in the analyst's own developmental project? Winnicott, with his characteristic tact, kept these questions in the background, and made due acknowledgement of the importance to him of Klein's contribution.

Winnicott uses this paper to describe a kind of bright child with 'a vivacity which immediately contributes something to one's mood, so that one feels lighter'.[74] He proposes that the lively child with the depressed mother is having to sustain the mother's vitality. He is keeping her alive as at least the semblance of a sentient presence. At the cost of his own needs, the child takes on both the mother's guilt and depression by identifying with it, and also the false but necessary solution of being blithe to cheer her up. The mother's depression is experienced by the child as an overriding demand that makes his own demands impossible. The risk is then that the child will, as Winnicott writes, 'use the mother's depression as an escape from his or her own'. The child who is lively is making reparation to the mother for something which he hasn't done and can't understand. And this makes it impossible for him to reach responsibility for his own impulses in relation to her. The relatively powerless infant and child can 'only accept the fact of mother's mood' – once again the father doesn't seem to come into the picture, everything being left to the child – and do what he can to meet it. There is, though, an absolute mismatch of preoccupation between mother and child. The child can, of course, exploit such a situation as another way of avoiding the pain of his own guilt. But Winnicott's main point in this paper is to stress that the child with a depressed mother can only live, to use a crucial Winnicottian term, *reactively*. He cannot initiate out of his own desire a gesture met by the mother but must always care for her in the hope that he will eventually establish the mother he needs to facilitate his own growth. If the children who have to deal first with their mother's mood 'succeed in the immediate task, they do no more than succeed', Winnicott writes, 'in creating an atmosphere in which they can *start on their own lives'*.[75]

Increasingly in his work now Winnicott took the ordinary development born of good-enough mothering as the norm and then set out to understand whatever interfered with it. At the very beginning life was problematic but not a form of illness. To make sense of psychopathology it was as if Winnicott was asking a simple question: given the infant's dependence on the mother, what resources were available to the infant and child that could make up for the deficits in the mothering he needed to sustain the continuity of his development? He found that the paradox of these childhood solutions was that they enabled the child to survive, but with the unconscious project and hope of finding an environment in which development could start up again. A life could be lived, that is to say, in suspended animation.

But the way a life was conceived of in psychoanalysis was determined by the fantasy of the very beginning. Klein, following Freud, believed in a primal and therefore formative ambivalence; Winnicott posited an original pre-ambivalent dependence. In fact his developmental story required, for its very beginning, a utopian idea. Utopian, that is to say, from the infant's point of view, and existing this side of the womb. 'Let us assume', he writes in one of his most distinctively original papers, 'The Mind and its Relation to the Psyche-Soma' (1949),[76]

that health in the early development of the individual entails continuity of being. The early psyche-soma proceeds along a certain line of development provided its continuity of being is not disturbed; in other words for the healthy development of the early psyche-soma there is a need for a perfect environment. At first the need is absolute. The perfect environment is one which actively adapts to the needs of the newly formed psyche-soma, that which we as observers know to be the infant at the start. A bad environment is bad because by failure to adapt it becomes an impingement to which the psyche-soma (i.e. the infant) must react. This reacting disturbs the continuity of the going on being of the individual.[77]

Birth can be the prototype for this impingement or interruption of the infant's going-on-being: 'during birth', Winnicott writes in 'Birth Memories, Birth Trauma, and Anxiety' (1949), 'the infant is a reactor.' As long as this reacting is not 'so powerful or so prolonged as to snap the thread of the infant's continuous process' he can, Winnicott believes, return to 'a state of not having to react, which is the only state in which the self can begin to be'.[78] The self can only grow in a state of protected unawareness because at the very earliest stages, Winnicott writes, 'there is not sufficient ego-strength for there to be a reaction without loss of identity'.[79] In Winnicott's terms psychopathology – and it could be recreated in an overdemanding analytic setting – was reaction as loss of identity, coping as a substitute for being. In Winnicott's description of this first stage of life a delicate and precarious process is described in which something impalpable but essential called the going-on-being of the infant can be ruptured if, as Winnicott says, 'an infant has to cope with an environment which insists on being important'.[80] The environment must be a medium without any demand that distracts the infant from his growth process. Whatever the infant cannot use for his development is – like a 'bad' interpretation in analysis – potentially an impingement. Having to deal with critical interruptions, like being woken by the phone in the middle of the night, involves a loss of continuity that Winnicott equates, at the earliest stage, with an emerging self. What Winnicott will call the False Self is habituated through early environmental

94

failure to living reactively; and may, in fact, busily 'collect impingements' – surround himself with demands – as a way of both trying to feel alive, and of turning what was once a passive experience into a more active one by demanding demands.

What Winnicott then refers to as the 'mind' can be used as part of the individual's primary project of finding the perfect environment. The environment that is the perfect medium for the True Self. 'In health,' Winnicott writes, with an eye on that other figure that preoccupied him, the Intellectual, 'the mind does not usurp the environment's function, but makes possible an understanding and eventually a making use of its relative failure.'[81] The mind is then, in a sense, continuous with, and can partly take over from, the environment. The child will mother himself or, rather, foster-mother himself with his mind. In terms of later development Winnicott suggests that 'in the care of an infant the mother is dependent on the infant's intellectual processes'.[82] It is noticeable that in this account the mind, in its rudimentary form, is a mother, a process of self-care based on mothering; there is not a paternal element, nor is there anywhere in Winnicott's work even an implied account of how a person fathers himself.

If the environmental failure is severe – beyond the infant's comprehension – then he will, in despair, develop a militant fantasy of self-sufficiency in which the mind will be used not to continue the mother's care but to displace it altogether. What Winnicott calls the psyche – a word oddly repressed in psychoanalysis, which Winnicott uses for that part of the body capable of mentation – becomes dissociated from the body and a kind of uprooted mental functioning evolves that is, Winnicott believes, 'an encumbrance to the psyche-soma or to the individual being's continuity of being which constitutes the self'.[83] The psyche attempts to disown the body which, due to maternal neglect, is felt to be a persecutor. What Winnicott calls 'excessive mental functioning' and wants to equate sometimes in this paper with the mind itself, is the infant's solution to 'erratic mothering'. What we conventionally refer to as the mind can be, in Winnicott's terms, a part of the personality born of tantalization; not integral to development but expedient. 'The true self,' he writes, 'a continuity of being, is in health based on psyche-soma growth . . . there is no localization of a mind self, and there is nothing that can be called a mind.'[84] The mind, given good-enough mothering, cannot be conceived of as a separate organ. Just as there was, for Winnicott, no such thing as a baby but only a nursing couple so, at best, there is no such thing as a mind, only a psyche-soma couple. And part of the function of the pathological split-off mind that Winnicott describes is to take on responsibility for an environment that failed. A genuine grievance about something in his early environment that the infant was incapable of modifying is turned against the self. The child lives as if there is no mother, an apparently self-sufficient unit located in the mind. So one of the aims of analysis would be to help the patient sort out environmental failure from that which he can genuinely take responsibility for as a part of himself. And this could involve the analyst, at times, in taking the patient's part against the parents. (Margaret Little recalled Winnicott saying to her, at one point in her analysis with him, 'I really *hate* your mother.'[85]) There are, of course, perils attached to Winnicott's position; in order to recognize a developmental distortion one must have a confident sense of what 'true' development consists of.

The end of the decade was a turbulent period in Winnicott's private life. In 1948 his father died and he suffered his first coronary. His marriage had for a long time been unhappy but he had felt unable to divorce his wife while his father was still alive. In 1949 he finally divorced Alice and

two years later married Clare Britton and began to establish
his own distinctive position in British psychoanalysis. In
the next twenty years he wrote most of the papers for which
he gained international recognition. But it is important to
realize, by way of conclusion, that during the 1940s Winnicott had evolved a powerful rival developmental theory to
those of both Freud and Klein, while including the bits of
their work he found useful. He was a pragmatist with an
essentialist theory that posited the existence of a True Self
that was rooted in the body, of a piece with it, so to speak,
but a body without erotic connotation. The drive was not
for pleasure but for development, and the foundations of
previous psychoanalytic theory – the Unconscious and the
Instincts – were subsumed by this project. The infant's life
began not exclusively in conflict but in mutuality; indeed
too much conflict distorted natural development. At the
earliest stages of development there was, as it were, a
rudimentary socialism, a form of life, Winnicott suggests,
based on collaborative exchange (or perhaps more exactly,
to use Wordsworth's phrase, 'mutual domination'). And so
by implication, in Winnicott's new-found terms, there were
parts of the Freudian and Kleinian developmental schema
that were descriptions, not of ordinary development, in his
view, but of the development of what he begins to call a
False Self. But there was one further paradox: Winnicott
was developing a negative theology of the Self in which the
True Self could not easily be described but only inferred to
be all that the False Self was not. It was to the elusiveness
of Selves and the creative truth of the body that Winnicott
was to devote the next twenty years of his work.

4 The Appearing Self

'Development itself is not an object that can be "desired".'

W. R. Bion

The papers Winnicott gave to non-psychoanalytic audiences are the best guide, at any given period, to his strongest convictions about psychoanalysis. In the papers collected in *The Family and Individual Development*, written between 1950 and 1962, he stressed the value of treating emotional problems by non-interference, by the provision of a holding environment in which 'natural' growth processes could reassert themselves. 'If we can adjust ourselves to these natural processes,' he writes, 'we can leave most of these complex mechanisms to nature, while we sit back and watch and learn.'[1] It is an 'if' of considerable importance in Winnicott's personal vision of the psychoanalytic cure. 'One general idea', he writes in a talk to midwives, 'goes right through what I have to say: that is that there are natural processes which underlie all that is taking place; and we do good work as doctors and nurses only if we respect and facilitate these natural processes.'[2] Winnicott could only convey indirectly, to these non-specialist audiences, his growing sense that a too militantly knowing psychoanalysis had usurped, or simply lacked confidence in, what he called 'essentially natural processes'. In these 'unofficial' papers and talks Klein and her followers were, albeit unbeknown to his various audiences, the objects of Winnicott's implicit

98

criticism. His belief in Nature had become, among other things, a covert critique of overinterpretative methods of psychoanalysis that had no faith in development as a natural human tendency. People could not be made to develop but they could be provided with a relatively unintrusive setting in which development was possible. 'As a psychoanalyst,' Winnicott wrote at this time, 'I have had very good training in this matter of waiting and waiting and waiting.'[3]

But were such 'natural processes' simple or complicated? What do we need to know about them in order to adjust to them when, in Winnicott's view, 'if parents have succeeded as parents they are unaware of the things in themselves that have made for success'?[4] On the one hand, in Winnicott's work of this period, he expresses a marked preference – that is often an idealization – for the 'silent integrative forces' of nature and the tacit knowledge or 'feeling attitude' of what he calls the 'ordinary devoted mother'. On the other hand he comes to increasingly complex and often obscure formulations about the earliest 'natural' stages of the infant's development that involve him in a radical revision of the kinds of instinct-theory that psychoanalysis had been traditionally based on. As we shall see, some of his most puzzling theoretical work becomes what Charles Rycroft has criticized as 'a personal statement, too idiosyncratic to be readily assimilated into the general body of any scientific theory'.[5] It is also fair to recognize that Winnicott had the psychoanalytic virtues of his scientific vices: he did not become systematically coherent at the cost of his own inventiveness.

It is in these last two decades of his life that Winnicott begins, quite explicitly, to separate himself from Klein, and, less explicitly, from Freud. His continued attentiveness over thirty years as both paediatrician and psychoanalyst to what mothers and their infants actually did together had changed his assumptions about what went on *inside* the infant. He

believed that Klein and her increasingly devoted followers
had described the infant in isolation from the actual reciprocal primary relationship in which he developed, and that,
rendering the mother anonymous, they had thereby over-
burdened the infant with innate characteristics. In her
influential paper of the decade, 'Envy and Gratitude' (1957),[6]
for example, Klein proposed that the infant was born
innately envious of the mother. For Winnicott envy was the
consequence of tantalizing mothering. It was constituted by
a certain kind of relationship and not a quasi-genetic characteristic. From his point of view Klein had been describing
not the ordinary developing infant but the failure of a
holding environment.

Winnicott was now more emphatic in his claim that in
Klein's work, 'the infant is not being directly observed, else
there must be a reference to the behaviour of the mother on
whom the infant is dependent. Id-relationships are only
meaningful to the infant if they happen in a framework of
Ego-relatedness.'[7] This was the conviction at the centre of
Winnicott's developmental theory. It was the rapport
between the mother and her infant that made instinctual
satisfaction possible; previous psychoanalytic theory had
assumed it was the other way round. This is why the apparently sophisticated notion of 'meaningfulness' replaces gratification as the main criterion of instinctual satisfaction in
Winnicott's account of the earliest relationship. Without this
rapport between the mother and her infant – what Winnicott
calls here 'Ego-relatedness' – the infant experiences his desire
as an overwhelming assault. The mother holds the experience
to make it satisfying. Where the Id of the infant is, there the
mother's Ego must be also.

So the 'good breast' of Kleinian jargon is not simply a
thing that arrives when the infant is hungry. In Winnicott's
terms it is not an object but a way of describing a process of
maternal care; it is, he writes, 'the name given to the

presenting of breast (or bottle) to the infant, a most delicate
affiar, and one which can only be done well enough at the
beginning if the mother is in a most curious state of
sensitivity which I (for the time being) call the State of
Primary Maternal Preoccupation'[8]. The infant's earliest
stages of development depend upon this notion of presentation, of the unimpinging attentive presence of the mother
and the ways in which she makes herself available in her
new state of being absorbed in her infant. The way the
breast was presented to the infant so that it seemed of a
piece with his desire was a paradigm, in Winnicott's terms,
of what the growing child would later be able to make of
the other objects he found in the world. The way the breast
was presented made desire presentable for the infant, en-
abling him to build up 'the basic stuff of the inner world
that is personal and indeed the self'. The mother makes
what is in fact a dialogue between her and her infant appear
to him as a monologue born of his desire. By virtue of the
mother's adaptation, as we have seen, there is an area of
illusion; it is as though, from the infant's point of view, he
creates in fantasy the mother he needs and finds. The infant,
in Winnicott's account, discovers the world by first creating
it; he is born an artist and a hedonist. Where Freud and
Klein had emphasized the role of disillusionment in human
development, in which growing up was a process of mourning, for Winnicott there was a more primary sense in which
development was a creative process of collaboration. Disillusionment presupposed sufficient illusionment. For the
infant at the very beginning, given a holding environment,
desire was creative rather than simply rapacious.

So, in an important review written with Masud Khan in
1953, Winnicott was critical of the work of the Scottish
psychoanalyst Ronald Fairbairn because it 'lines up with
theory given us by Melanie Klein which also allows no
tribute to be paid to the idea of primary psychic creativity'.[9]

In what they refer to as 'strictly Freudian theory' concerned with the 'instinctual elements' of relationships,

> no claim is being made that these matters cover the entire range of human experience. It would seem that only comparatively recently have analysts begun to feel the need for a hypothesis that would allow for areas of infancy experience and of ego-development that are not basically associated with instinctual conflict and where there is instrinsically a psychic process such as that which we have here termed 'primary (psychic) creativity'.[10]

The fundamental psychoanalytic questions being addressed here are twofold: first, does instinctual life at its earliest stages necessarily imply conflict? And secondly, what does an account of human experience based on the notion of instinctual conflict leave out? It was the Independent or Middle Group that was emerging in the British Society in the 1950s that felt the need for a revisionary hypothesis that provided ways of answering these questions. And the questions themselves, of course, and the idea of 'primary psychic creativity', were radically at odds with the Freudian model. In Freud's work creativity was the (mostly adult) sublimation of infantile sexuality, though he never gave a convincing account of the actual nature of sublimatory activity itself. For Melanie Klein creativity as essentially reparative – for Klein, art *was* reparation – was secondary to the destructiveness inherent in infantile sexuality as witnessed by the infant himself in the depressive position. In Winnicott's new theory, creativity was primary, pre-sexual, and characterized the naturally reciprocal relationship of a baby and his 'ordinary devoted mother'.

If early development was literally creative – the infant creating out of desire the mother who is ready to be found – then he begins with an absolute claim on her. Through her Primary Preoccupation with his well-being it is as though she belongs to him. But in time the unconditional nature of the claim changes. As the infant grows from a state of absolute dependence on the mother to a state of relative dependence, and the mother begins to emerge from her Primary Maternal Preoccupation, the infant begins to experience disillusionment. Optimally the mother's continuing adaptation to her infant ensures that these recurring experiences are within the range of his (growing) tolerance. If they are not, if he feels traumatically let down by her, he may eventually begin to steal as a way of symbolically reasserting his earliest claim on her. But the stealing itself, as Winnicott had realized in his work with evacuated children during the war, was an affirmation that the child had once had good early experiences that had been disrupted. In the 1950s Winnicott tried to give a more detailed and coherent account of these processes. If the 'area of illusion' has been established between mother and infant, how does the infant go on to include in his life other Not-Me objects? Or, to ask the question in a different way, how does the infant make the transition from being merged in with the mother to being separate? What is the mother's role in these processes, and what symptomatology will the child use to restore the continuity of his life if the environment fails him? In three of the most important papers of the decade – 'Primary Maternal Preoccupation' (1956),[11] 'The Anti-Social Tendency' (1956),[12] and 'Transitional Objects and Transitional Phenomena' (1951)[13] – Winnicott addressed these issues. But behind his interest in these subjects there was, to borrow the title of another of his seminal papers, 'Aggression in Relation to Emotional Development'.[14] It was the nature of aggression and its role in development that consistently perplexed him. It was clearly integral to the process of personal individuation, and yet it was not obviously an instinct that was comparable to the sexual instinct. It was the subject, as we shall see, of his most powerful insights and his most opaque formulations. And it was to be through his understanding of aggression that Winnicott would finally separate himself from Klein.

II

Reviewing a book called *Aggression and its Interpretation* for the *British Medical Journal*, Winnicott suggested, in a paragraph marked by its brevity, that, 'An intuitive flash of the author quite possibly goes very deep: "the primary, powerful innate urge to self-realization as the basis of aggression".'[15] It was unusual at this time – 1954 – for a psychoanalyst to value either intuitive flashes or notions of *self*-realization. In psychoanalysis, instincts had their vicissitudes and destinies but not selves. Melanie Klein, developing Freud's later idea of a Death instinct, proposed a theory that, as we have seen, took for granted an innate destructiveness in the infant that she often simply called 'hate' and which was opposed, in stark allegorical simplicity, to 'love'. Winnicott considered the idea of a Death *instinct* a misnomer and Klein's use of the word 'hate' a misleading oversimplification.[16] In relation to what Masud Khan has called Winnicott's 'humane empiricism', these beliefs were baggy abstractions based on insufficient observation. 'Aggression' was not one thing, and the purposes it served in individual development changed over time. In three papers written during the 1950s – 'Aggression in Relation to Emotional Development' (1950),[17] 'The Depressive Position and Normal Development' (1954),[18] and 'Psychoanalysis and the Sense of Guilt' (1957)[19] – Winnicott tried to replace Klein's vocabulary – which, in his view, had pathologized ordinary development – with a natural history of the role of aggression in emotional development. Winnicott is most distinctively himself when summarizing his ideas for a non-specialist audience. In a paper written for doctors in 1958, with the subtitle 'Modern Views on Emotional Development', he claims that 'motility is the precursor of aggression, which is a term that develops meaning as the infant grows'.[20] There was, he believed, an innate developmental energy that had a specifically aggressive quality and could be used to describe the movements of the foetus, the baby's hand grasp, and the chewing activities that would eventually turn into biting. In health this 'aggressive potential' is mostly 'fused in with the infant's instinctual experiences, and with the pattern of the individual infant's relationships'. But, in illness, Winnicott writes,

> only a small proportion of the aggressive potential becomes fused in with the erotic life, and the infant is then burdened with impulses that make no sense. These eventually lead to destructiveness in the relationship to objects, or, worse, form the basis of activity that is entirely senseless, as, for instance, a convulsion.[21]

This 'aggressive potential' that is not referred to as an instinct is tantamount, in Winnicott's writing of this period, to a developmental potential. 'Aggression', he writes elsewhere, 'is seen more as evidence of life.'[22] But it has to be included, 'fused in', with the infant's capacity for instinctual relationship that he equates with the 'erotic life' of the infant. They are, he makes clear, separate forces that need to be fused and brought into relation with an object. Otherwise this aggressive potential might be dissociated or experienced as an alien force in the personality. Destructiveness is aggression unmodified by relationship;

it makes no sense if it exists in isolation, in a context in which sense cannot be made of it. But it is important to note that in this account what Winnicott calls instincts are insufficient in themselves, without the aggressive potential, for the infant's full development. And the relationship between the 'erotic life' and the 'aggressive potential' is one of mutual dependence. This is, of course, quite different from Freud's (and Klein's) view of development as what Freud called 'the struggle between Eros and Death'.[23] From a more orthodox psychoanalytic point of view, Winnicott's terms were potentially confusing. For the British Society the interesting muddles that attend the difficult questions had to be turned into something more schematic, if only to provide opportunity for discussion.

In 'Aggression in Relation to Emotional Development' Winnicott attempted to provide his own normative sequence in which he postulated a primary aggression that was neither an instinct nor synonymous with any urge for destruction. 'Prior to integration of the personality,' he writes, 'there is aggression' and 'an original aggressiveness is almost synonymous with activity'. What we call aggression only makes sense when 'aggression is meant', but this in itself is a developmental achievement. If, at the very beginning, a baby chews the nipple, in Winnicott's view – and here he implicitly disagrees with Klein – 'it cannot be assumed that he is meaning to destroy or hurt'. To believe this would be to inflict intentions on the infant of precocious sophistication. Aggression at the beginning of life is, for Winnicott, 'part of the primitive expression of love . . . the primitive love impulse (id) has a destructive quality, though it is not the infant's aim to destroy since the impulse is experienced in the pre-ruth era'.[24] At the first stage of development, that is pre-integration, aggression is part of the infant's natural appetite, what Winnicott calls 'purpose without concern' in which the infant's 'excited love includes an imaginative attack on the mother's body'. He proposes a 'theoretical stage of unconcern or ruthlessness in which the child can be said to exist as a person and to have purpose, yet to be unconcerned as to results'.[25] From the infant's point of view he cannot be described as hating or wishing to destroy the mother at this stage but only as carelessly loving her. It is a theory, then, not of Original Sin but of what might be called Original Ruthless Virtue. The stage of unconcern, related as it was in Winnicott's mind to primary psychic creativity, was becoming one of his main theoretical preoccupations.

At the next stage, owing to the infant's integration, instincts can begin to be owned as personal intentions. The infant becomes aware of an inside and an outside and a mother who is outside as a source of nourishment and comfort. Acknowledging the mother as the object of his desire, the infant becomes concerned for her welfare and the damage his desire might do her. What Klein had described as the Depressive Position, Winnicott renames the Stage of Concern; something sounding ominously like a psychiatric syndrome becomes a more ordinarily recognizable feeling. This stage brings with it 'the capacity to feel guilty' and therefore feelings that now can be more accurately described as anger. But all this does require the attentive collaboration of the mother. From Winnicott's point of view, Klein, in her description of the depressive position had failed to include the mother's role in which, over a long period of time, she 'holds a situation so that the infant has the chance to work through the consequences of instinctual experiences'.[26] In 'Psychoanalysis and the Sense of Guilt' he refers to the 'innumerable repetitions spread over a period of time' of what he calls the 'benign circle' that constitutes the stage of concern: '(1) instinctual experience, (2) acceptance of responsibility (by the infant), which is called guilt, (3) a working through, and (4) a true restitutive gesture.'[27] This benign circle relies on the mother's responsiveness in a way that Klein never stressed. It depends, Winnicott writes, 'on the mother's capacity to survive the instinctual moment, and so to be there to receive and understand the true reparative gesture'.[28] Only then is the infant able 'to accept responsibility for the total phantasy of the full instinctual impulse that was previously ruthless. Ruthlessness gives way to ruth, unconcern to concern.'[29] The infant becomes able to imagine and so to connect the object of desire – what Winnicott will call the Object Mother – with the object of more general care – the Environment Mother. And by the same process he will connect himself as a desiring person with the more quiescent and comfortable person he is between feeds. The baby, as Winnicott says, 'puts one and one together and begins to see that the answer is one, and not two'.[30]

But it should be noticed that Winnicott is proposing a quite different picture of the origins of the infant's desire: in Klein's account, in the earliest paranoid-schizoid position (that Winnicott finds no use for), the infant was described, we may remember, as actively splitting the mother into a good breast and a bad breast. The depressive position was the developmentally necessary attempt to heal the split, to bring together the destructive instincts with the loving instincts in relation to what in actuality was one mother. Winnicott proposes a pre-fusion, pre-integration 'era' consisting of what he variously calls 'aggressive potential' or 'aggressive components' and erotic instincts. Optimally these become fused in the primitive love impulse in relation to the Object Mother of desire. While the Kleinian infant at the earliest stages cannot link the good breast and the bad breast, the Winnicottian infant cannot link the mother he eats with the mother who cares for him in a more general way between feeds. But Winnicott still has to account for what he calls the pre-fusion era in which the primitive love impulse is constituted by the fusion of an aggressive component and an erotic instinct. 'Proper significance', he writes, 'has not been given in psychoanalytic theory to the pre-fusion era and the task of fusion.'[31]

In his clinical work with regressed patients, he reports becoming aware that 'when a patient is engaged in discovering the aggressive root the analyst is more exhausted by the process, one way or another, than when the patient is discovering the erotic root of the instinctual life'.[32] He implies in this passage that there are two 'roots' to instinctual life, but not two instincts. He has found that the aggressive and erotic 'components' involve the object in significantly different kinds of relationship. 'The erotic experiences can be completed while the object is subjectively conceived or personally created';[33] the hungry infant fantasizes a satisfying object which by its timely arrival appears to belong to him as his own creation. But it is through the aggressive component, Winnicott suggests, that the infant establishes the existence of a separate external world, a world that by resisting him affords him the definition of his own limits. 'In the early stages,' Winnicott writes, 'when the Me and the Not-Me are being established, it is the aggressive component that more surely drives the individual to a need for a Not-Me or an object that is felt to be external.'[34] Winnicott is close to saying here that there is an innate agonistic tendency in the developing infant. While the erotic components seek their complementary satisfaction from an object not necessarily experienced as other, the aggressive component invites opposition; indeed, 'the aggressive impulses do not give any satisfactory experience unless there is opposition'. Through the erotic component at the early stages the infant and the object of his desire are seemingly identical;

the aggressive component satisfies a desire for differentiation. The aggressive component require external opposition to make development possible, but when opposition is excessive it turns into impingement and then, Winnicott writes, 'the life-force is taken up in reactions to impingement'. It should be obvious by now that as Winnicott initiates important distinctions he also changes terminology in a confusing way; in the above quotations aggressive 'components' have become 'impulses' and 'instinctual life' has turned into 'the life-force'. All these terms have quite different implications.

Elaborating this fundamental distinction between the erotic and the aggressive, Winnicott reports that 'patients let us know that the aggressive experiences (more or less defused) feel real, much more real than do the erotic experiences (also defused)'.[35] 'Real' here means that the patient feels contact has been made with something genuinely other that resists coercion. There is a distinct shift of register from psychoanalytic formulation to the ordinary language of patients and a vocabulary concerned with the quality of experience. Winnicott goes on to assert that 'each baby has a potential of zonal erotic instinct, that this is biological, and that the potential is more or less the same for each baby. By contrast the aggression component must be extremely variable.'[36] The aggression is variable because it depends on the opposition given by the environment, the way limits are set to movement, or other bodily expression. It is the amount of opposition that 'affects the conversion of life-force into aggression potential'. But it is difficult to see how Winnicott could know that the potential of erotic instinct is the same in everyone. It is as though, he assumes, the erotic life is a great leveller.

Winnicott is proposing that an initially unified 'life-force' splits in the earliest stages of development into two components: the aggressive component, born of opposition, and the erotic component, born of complementarity. 'Real' in this idiosyncratic system comes to mean distinct; 'unreal', by implication the realm of the erotic, means at least partly merged in with. It is therefore only through the aggressive component that relationship with real others can exist. There is in Winnicott's account of the early pre-fused era a distrust of the erotic and a curiously idealized nostalgia for the unfused ruthlessly aggressive component, and this leads him to a puzzling formulation which is, he says,

> a description of the common state in which *some degree of lack of fusion* has been a feature. The personality comprises three parts: a true self, with Me and Not-Me clearly established, and with some fusion of the aggressive and erotic elements; a self that is easily seduced along lines of erotic experience, but with the result of a loss of sense of real; a self that is entirely and ruthlessly given over to aggression.[37]

In this tripartite model – which Winnicott does not use again – of the personality constituted by multiple selves, it is the third one that he refers to as having 'value to the individual because it brings a sense of real and a sense of relating'. Although the fusion of the aggression and the erotic component (now called 'elements') in the true self 'enhances the feeling of the reality of the experience', it is nevertheless represented here by Winnicott as something of a compromise. Vitality and the sense of being really alive are clearly bound up for him with the aggressive component. In fact, he goes on to suggest that what we refer to as aggression is sometimes more accurately described as spontaneity, for Winnicott the cardinal virtue of the good life. The 'life-force', as expressed by the 'impulsive gesture', he writes,

> becomes aggressive when opposition is reached. There is reality in this experience, and it very easily fuses

into the erotic experiences that await the new-born infant. I am suggesting: *it is this impulsiveness, and the aggression that develops out of it, that makes the infant need an external object,* and not merely a satisfying object.[38]

The impulsive gesture must be met, but the infant needs in the mother a collaborator – at once sufficiently other, and sufficiently identified with him – but not an accomplice. It is the responsive opposition of the external object that facilitates the aggression necessary for development. And Winnicott explained, in the papers we have been looking at, the way in which instinctual satisfaction was potentially annihilating for the infant who becomes distressed if 'physical satisfaction too quickly robs [him] of zest. The infant is then left with: aggression undischarged – because not enough muscle erotism or primitive impulse (or motility) was used in the feeding process.'[39] It is the aggressive component that makes whole-hearted instinctual experience possible, and which has also to be met by the mother. Winnicott was now beginning to equate creativity not with the relatively late stage of reparation and concern but with the primitive love impulse, the whole-hearted earliest instinctual experiences which included an aggressive ruthlessness.

In earlier papers Winnicott had made brief and provocative reference to his dissatisfaction with the Kleinian view of creativity.[40] The Kleinian aesthetic was in the ascendant in the British Society but as early as 1948 Winnicott had suggested in a single and sufficiently oblique sentence that 'there were other roots for creativeness but reparation provides an important link between the creative impulse and the life the patient leads'.[41] In 'The Depressive Position in Normal Emotional Development' he wrote that guilt and the consequent wish to make reparation were 'one source

of potency and social contribution, and of artistic performance (but not of art itself which has roots at a deeper
level)'.[42] But in 'Psychoanalysis and the Sense of Guilt' he
makes quite explicit his view that creativity is bound up
with a capacity for ruthlessness. 'The creative artist or
thinker', he writes, 'may, in fact, fail to understand, or even
may despise, the feelings of concern that motivate a less
creative person.' It is the artist's ruthlessness that 'does in
fact . . . achieve more than guilt-driven labour'.[43] Reparation
could be a flight from inspiration.

For Winnicott, then, the very earliest stages of development were intrinsically creative; and creativity was bound
up with the third self in the personality 'entirely and
ruthlessly given over to aggression'. And integral to development and creativity alike was the search for an object,
or an environment, or a medium, sufficiently resilient and
responsive to withstand the full blast of the primitive love
impulse. In Winnicott's later work, as we shall see, he
takes up these issues again.

But if the provision of a good-enough early environment
could be taken for granted, if primary creativity and a
capacity for illusionment were established facts of the
infant's development, how did the infant and child eventually reach a stage of relative independence? Winnicott
would answer this question from a simple observation that
generated his most celebrated concept: it was, he realized,
via the infant's use of his first Not-Me object, which
Winnicott called a transitional object.

II

Winnicott saw the infant's gradual differentiation from the
mother as a process of transition from absolute dependence
on her as an object subjectively conceived – the desired
breast found when imagined by the hungry infant as though

113

by magic – towards relative independence of, and relationship with, an object discovered to be beyond omnipotent control. The infant developed from a state of pure subjectivity to a capacity for virtual objectivity that Winnicott associated with scientific method. But the kind of science he valued had its roots, he insisted, in the more primitive states of subjectivity out of which it had grown and on which it depended. Development was not progressive mastery, an overcoming of earlier stages, but a process of inclusive combination. There was always a risk, for example, that 'those who are most reliably objective are often comparatively out of touch with their own inner world's richness'.[44] What Winnicott called Transitional Phenomena made possible for the child these early fundamental transitions from subjectivity to objectivity, from being merged in with the mother to being also separate from her. The Transitional Phenomena that provided a bridge between the inner and outer worlds gave continuity to a process where previously, from a psychoanalytic point of view, there seemed to be only mutually exclusive options: either subjectivity or objectivity, either unity with the mother or separateness, either invention or discovery. The Transitional Object is always a combination, but one that provides, by virtue of being more than the sum of its parts, a new, third alternative. And it is never merely a substitute for something else.

In the spatula game Winnicott had noted the infant's early use of what he called a Not-Me possession. In his influential paper 'Transitional Objects and Transitional Phenomena',[45] he extends this idea that 'sooner or later in an infant's development there comes a tendency on the part of the infant to weave other-than-me objects into the personal pattern'.[46] Woven in, they become an addition to an already existing pattern. Most children, quite early on, find for themselves a special and unshareable object – a teddy-bear, a particular doll or toy, a piece of material – that is, for a time, indispensable to them. By definition this object cannot be imposed on the child; though it may have been given him, it cannot be given him as a Transitional Object, but only as something he may choose to turn into one. In the same way a good interpretation in analysis cannot be given to a patient: it can only be found by him to be so ('meaning', unlike information, cannot be imposed, but only found through personal recognition). Winnicott suggests that there is a continuity between the child's use of this first object and the adult's later use of the cultural tradition as it becomes meaningful to him. But unlike later and more sophisticated cultural objects, like works of art, the first Transitional Object is essentially idiosyncratic and unshareable. Winnicott, however, never makes clear how the child gets from the private experience to the more communal experience, from a personal teddy-bear to a pleasure in reading Dickens.

The first Transitional Object is defined by the kind of use the infant makes of it rather than by any more obviously shareable characteristics it is assumed, by an outsider, to possess. There is, he stresses, in this relationship to the first object, 'something . . . important here other than oral excitement and satisfaction, although this may be the basis of everything else'. It is worth quoting in full Winnicott's summary of the 'special qualities in the relationship':

1. The infant assumes rights over the object, and we agree to this assumption. Nevertheless some abrogation of omnipotence is a feature from the start.

2. The object is affectionately cuddled as well as excitedly loved and mutilated.

3. It must never change, unless changed by the infant.

4. It must survive instinctual loving, and also hating, and, if it be a feature, pure aggression.

115

5. Yet it must seem to the infant to give warmth, or to move, or to have texture, or to do something that seems to show it has vitality or reality of its own.

6. It comes from without from our point of view, but not so from the point of view of the baby. Neither does it come from within; it is not an hallucination.

7. Its fate is to be gradually allowed to be decathected, so that in the course of years it becomes not so much forgotten as relegated to limbo. By this I mean that in health the transitional object does not 'go inside' nor does the feeling about it necessarily undergo repression. It is not forgotten and it is not mourned. It loses meaning, and this is because the transitional phenomena have become diffused, have become spread out over the whole intermediate territory between 'inner psychic reality' and 'the external world as perceived by two persons in common', that is to say, over the whole cultural field.[47]

There is an overlap between those qualities the infant perceives as belonging to the mother and the qualities of this first Not-Me object. It has permanence, resilience and a degree of apparent autonomy. It is observable by others – 'not an hallucination' – but cannot have a comparable significance for them. And the affection with which the object is cuddled can be seen as the infant's way of linking the object-mother and the environment-mother. (Affection, and Winnicott's other transitional concept, 'spontaneity', are central to his new theory of object-relations.) But it is in the final section of his summary that the Transitional Object becomes a unique object in psychoanalytic discourse. Unlike every other object that figures in psychoanalysis it is neither lost nor internalized; it is not a substitute for anything else, anything prior, nor is it in turn substituted (though Limbo, we may remember, was on the border of

Hell). The object is part of a potential continuum of meaningful objects 'spread out over' the intermediate territory that for Winnicott constitutes what he calls the 'cultural field'; the Transitional Object eventually becomes merely irrelevant because there is a 'diffusion' – not a displacement – of significance; interest is dispersed into other things. But Winnicott's account, as I have said, tells us nothing about how or why new objects are selected; the cultural field is curiously undifferentiated. And his description is made difficult to imagine because his terms shift: diffusion is different from spreading out over. So it is still worth pressing the question, what does the infant use this object to do for him? In a paper written in the same year as his paper on Transitional Phenomena, Winnicott gives the recognizable example of the child who takes some precious object to bed with him at night:

> I call this thing a transitional object. By this means I can illustrate the one difficulty every child experiences is to relate subjective reality to shared reality which can be objectively perceived. From waking to sleeping the child jumps from a perceived world to a self-created world. In between there is a need for all kinds of transitional phenomena – neutral territory ... there is a tacit understanding that no one will claim that this real thing is a part of the world or that it is created by the infant. It is understood that both these things are true: the infant created and the world provided it. This is the continuation forward of the initial task which the ordinary mother enables her infant to undertake, when by a most delicate active adaptation she offers herself, perhaps her breast, a thousand times at the moment that the baby is ready to create something like the breast that she offers.[48]

The Transitional Object is here a bridge where otherwise the child would have to jump; and it bridges for the child what might seem, without this connection, to be two incompatible worlds. Similarly, at the other end of the process, when the child's dreaming experience, that most subjective inner reality, is represented in language and reported to someone, the dream enters what Winnicott calls here the 'neutral territory' or intermediate space of shared language. The child uses the bedtime object to reach to and connect the sleeping self that dreams and the waking self that can 'join in'. It makes possible one of the child's most fundamental transitions from waking to sleeping, just as in his account of the spatula game Winnicott had described that other fundamental transition from quiescence to desire. And it is what the child uses the object to do – here convey him safely from waking to sleeping – that interests Winnicott, not the specific nature of the object. And this idea could, of course, be extended to the analytic situation; in understanding the patient's transference at any given moment in the treatment the analyst might ask himself not only 'Who am I representing?' (mother, father, sibling, etc.), but also 'What am I being used to do?' The patient, in Winnicott's terms, is always trying to go somewhere via the analyst. Interpretations are passports.

The analytic setting itself could be seen as a transitional space for collaborative exchange. Prior to Winnicott's conceptualizing of all that was transitional in human experience, psychoanalysis, broadly speaking, had been a theory of subjects in some kind of instinctual relation to objects. From Winnicott's point of view, it had not taken sufficient notice of the space between them, except as an obstacle. In this space, desire crystallized; the fantasized wish to merge with or annihilate the object was an attempt to pre-empt the space, and a capacity to mourn the object constituted the space as real. But this space was also used by children to play in. Children's play was not only the child's more or less disguised representation of a craving for the object, but the child's finding and becoming a self. The transitional space in which the child plays, or the adult talks, is, in Winnicott's view, 'an intermediate area of *experiencing* to which inner reality and external life both contribute', and it exists as 'a resting-place for the individual engaged in the perpetual task of keeping inner and outer reality separate yet inter-related'.[49] Transitional space breaks down when either inner or outer reality begins to dominate the scene, just as a conversation stops if one of the participants takes over. At the very beginning, when the infant begins to be able to acknowledge that his monologue is, in fact, a dialogue, he needs this 'intermediate state between [his] inability and growing ability to recognize and accept reality', what Winnicott now refers to in the terms of his own developmental theory as 'the substance of illusion, that which is allowed to the infant, and which in adult life is inherent in art and religion'.[50] This is a long way from Freud's view of culture as the sublimation of instinctual life, or the wishful compensation for the frustrations imposed by reality. In the Freudian scheme, culture signifies instinctual renunciation; for Winnicott it was the only medium for self-realization.

What Winnicott rather misleadingly calls 'shared reality' is constituted by the sharing of illusions. Shared reality is the area of overlap between those individual preoccupations that Winnicott calls illusions, not because they are false but because they combine the desired with the actual in tolerable ways. 'If we wish,' he writes, 'we may collect together and form a group on the basis of the similarity of our illusory experiences. This is a natural root of grouping among human beings.'[51] Again, it is important to remember the original audience of the paper – the then divided British Society. In his quietly scandalous paper, Winnicott was

119

questioning not only the status of psychoanalytic theories
and institutions as Transitional Phenomena but also the
notion of psychoanalysis as a dogma he increasingly associated with the group around Klein. 'It is a hallmark of
madness', he goes on, 'when an adult puts too powerful a
claim on the credulity of others, forcing them to acknowledge the sharing of illusion that is not their own.'[52] Winnicott does not examine the question of what makes an
illusion shareable, or why, in psychoanalysis for example,
one story or set of explanations is convincing or satisfying
to some people and not others. What he does make clear is
that in his view there is something pathological about the
need to be believed. And this could be understood in
developmental terms; if the mother impinges on the infant
with her own desire and so does not allow him opportunity
for illusion, he can only comply with her, in order to
survive. For Winnicott it will be his notion of the False Self
that will be used by the child to manage the burden of the
imposed illusion that is not his own; the child, he writes in
a suggestive analogy, 'presents a shop-window or out-turned
half'.[53] It was in his important paper 'Primary Maternal
Preoccupation' that Winnicott described the conditions in
which the True Self came alive.

There is, however, one further thing that should be said
about this most famous of Winnicott's papers, 'Transitional
Objects and Transitional Phenomena'. It is noticeable that
as Winnicott tries to integrate his new idea into already
existing psychoanalytic theory he becomes confusing and
even self-contradictory. But he is exploring, from a psychoanalytic perspective, how a new object gets into the
orbit of the infant's interest; and the paper, in a sense,
enacts the problem it attempts to describe. It shows, in the
way the paper tells the story, both the fate of the new idea
in psychoanalysis, and the difficulty of conceiving, in psychoanalytic discourse, the manner in which a new object

ever enters a person's life without being exclusively a substitute for the primary object.

III

In 1956 Winnicott became President of the British Psychoanalytical Society and wrote two complementary papers – 'The Anti-Social Tendency' and 'Primary Maternal Preoccupation'[54] – which were both summings-up of work done during the war and attempts to formulate his own distinctive contribution. In his inaugural paper on Transitional Phenomena, published at the beginning of the decade, he had stated firmly that 'the mother's eventual task is gradually to disillusion the infant, but she has no hope of success unless at first she has been able to give sufficient opportunity for illusion'.[55] 'Illusion' was initially the infant's belief that he had created what he had in fact found. If he has established this belief, if the mother has fitted in with his desire, he has been, in Winnicott's terms, 'started off well enough by the mother' and so could use 'the intermediate area . . . that is allowed to the infant between primary creativity and objective perception based on reality testing'.[56] Transitional Phenomena provided a non-compliant solution to the infant's loss of omnipotence. It was disillusioning for the infant to discover the mother as real and beyond magical control. But development through the use of Transitional Phenomena was not for Winnicott, as it was for Freud, a process of cumulative disillusionment; it was not a growing capacity for mourning, but a growing capacity to tolerate the continual and increasingly sophisticated illusionment–disillusionment–re-illusionment process throughout the life-cycle. Weaning was then one of the serious, formative disillusionments in a series that had begun with the infant's primary creativity that the mother gradually modifies with what Winnicott calls 'doses' of reality.[57] 'It is assumed', Winnicott writes, 'that the task of reality acceptance is never completed, that no human being is free from the strain of relating inner and outer reality.'[58] It is through the use of Transitional Phenomena, the intermediate area, that the infant and later the adult are sustained between two impossible alternatives – the isolation and madness of excessive subjectivity or the impoverishment and anonymous futility of objectivity (or compliance masquerading as objectivity). In 'Primary Maternal Preoccupation' Winnicott describes the kind of environmental care that is required to make the intense subjectivity of early instinctual experience an enrichment of the self rather than merely a gratification of the organism. Winnicott intended, he said, to rescue the 'study of the mother from the purely biological'.

For Winnicott, primary maternal preoccupation was a state comparable to an illness and characterized by a preoccupation that began before birth and lasted for a few weeks after birth. It was a state of 'heightened sensitivity' akin to a kind of primitive, somatic identification with the baby. Anything that interfered with this earliest relationship was a dangerous interruption, and in Winnicott's view created an 'early distortion' of the infant's 'line of life', his 'going on being'. The image is of something inviolate growing through the quality of the attention it receives. Winnicott regards this as the normal state of 'an ordinary devoted mother' and the paradigm for later states of imaginative empathy. The infant's going on being is sustained by the mother's continued preoccupation. What Winnicott calls 'maternal failures' produce 'phases of reaction to impingement and these reactions interrupt the "going on being" of the infant. An excess of this reacting produces not frustration but a *threat of annihilation* ... a very real primitive anxiety, long antedating any anxiety that includes the word death in its description.'[59] What Freud and – following him – Klein had ascribed to the working of an innate Death instinct Winnicott again sees as a failure of the holding environment. The inattentive or absent mother is, in Winnicott's view, a saboteur of the developmental process that he equates with the continuity of care. Though not blaming mothers for their 'failures', he was implicitly demanding everything of them at the very beginning. 'Only if a mother is sensitized in the way I am describing', he writes with unusually dogmatic conviction, 'can she feel herself into her infant's place and so meet the infant's needs.'[60]

But it is the nature of the infant's needs that is in question. Psychoanalysis, of course, has an array of terms – instincts, needs, wishes, demands, desires, elements, components, drives – all of which refer to the imperious parts of the self. And it is the imperious parts of the self that are conceived to be essential. Freud was always committed to a dual instinct theory, and up until the early 1920s distinguished between 'ego-instincts', that were self-preservative, and sexual instincts. These were considerably modified and replaced in his later work by Life and Death instincts, which were, as we have seen, the foundation of Klein's work. Winnicott, as usual playing fast and loose with psychoanalytic terminology, suggests that for the infant there are 'at first body-needs, and they gradually become ego-needs as a psychology emerges out of the imaginative elaboration of physical experience'.[61] Winnicott is proposing here, not a conflict between different kinds of instinct, but a metamorphosis of one kind of 'need' into another. Resisting the limitation of definitions, Winnicott's sometimes confusing personal idiom often depends on the reader getting a sense of what he means. Here ego-needs, like a 'psychology', are a growing conscious awareness – an imaginative elaboration – on the part of the child of the repertoire of his developmental needs. Winnicott believed that psychoanalysis had never worked out the connection between instincts on the one hand and an individual's developmental tendency on the other. For Winnicott the developmental tendency was not constituted by the instincts but served by them. The mother's primary maternal preoccupation at the beginning

> provides a setting for the infant's constitution to begin to make itself evident, for the developmental tendencies to start to unfold, and for the infant to experience spontaneous movement and become the owner of the sensations that are appropriate to this early phase of life. The instinctual life need not be referred to here because what I am discussing begins before the establishment of instinct patterns.[62]

For Winnicott the analytic situation replicates the setting he describes, the analyst being responsive through mostly verbalized recognition of the patient's developmental tendencies. The earliest stages of development are seen as a process of unfolding (the analogy again with plant life) and self-appropriation of the disarray of sensation and motility held together by the conducive milieu of maternal care. What can be described as 'instinct patterns' can be constituted, in any meaningful sense, only in relation to the mother. The consistency of the mother's care as medium for growth 'enables the infant to begin to exist, to have experience, to build a personal ego, to ride instincts, and to meet with all the difficulties inherent in life. All this feels real to the infant who becomes able to have a self.'[63] This is a way of describing the integrity of the personality; if the early environment is sufficiently adaptive to what Winnicott calls 'constitutional factors', the individual's real idiosyncrasy is 'more likely to show up'. But in this paper in which he is beginning to need a self concept, Winnicott is insistent that if the mother is not sufficiently adaptive and demands of the infant a precocious adaptation to her own needs,

> The feeling of real is absent and if there is not too much chaos the ultimate feeling is of futility. The inherent difficulties of life cannot be reached, let alone the satisfactions. If there is not chaos there appears a false self that hides the true self, that complies with demands, that reacts to stimuli, that rids itself of instinctual experiences by having them, but that is only playing for time.[64]

The false self is playing for time until a sufficiently nurturing environment can be found in which development can start up again. Winnicott was beginning to see the individual's symptomatology as his way of representing not only or necessarily instinctual conflict – a developmental achievement in itself – but also the invisible history of the failures of mothering that had interrupted the continuity of his growth. Psychoanalysis would be a collaborative attempt to reconstruct the ways in which the mother in actuality, from the child's point of view, had failed the child; it would involve, that is to say, the locating of legitimate grievances.

It was no longer sexuality or the Death instinct that constituted the unacceptable in Winnicott's version of psychoanalysis, it was early dependence and the terrors involved, both in its full acknowledgement and in its possible insufficiency. This 'general failure of recognition', he writes, 'of absolute dependence at the start contributes to the fear of WOMAN that is the lot of both men and women.'[65] In the Postscript to his first collection of broadcast talks, published in 1957, Winnicott formulated what was, in effect, his sense of personal vocation:

> I suppose that everyone has a paramount interest, a deep, driving propulsion towards something. If one's

life lasts long enough, so that looking back becomes allowable, one discerns an urgent tendency that has integrated all the various and varied activities of one's private life and one's professional career. As for me I can already see what a big part has been played in my work by the urge to find and to appreciate the ordinary good mother ... for me it has been to mothers that I have so deeply needed to speak.'[66]

It is an uncharacteristically pious moment in Winnicott's writing. But he is, of course, describing a destiny vulnerable to those particular ironies that Freud's work makes possible.

5 Real-making

'Impeded aggressiveness seems to involve a
grave injury.'

Sigmund Freud

'We have yet to tackle the question', Winnicott wrote in
one of his last published papers, 'The Location of Cultural
Experience' (1967), 'of *what life itself is about.*'[1] It was the
large question, Winnicott believed, that psychoanalysts
seemed to have ignored, but that psychotic patients 'force
us to give attention to'. And in the last years of his life
Winnicott answered the question with a necessary kind of
elusiveness. He proposed an essentialist theory but with an
essence, the True Self, that by definition could not be
formulated except in the most rudimentary terms. 'It does
no more', he wrote, 'than collect together the details of the
experience of aliveness.'[2] Minimal definition allowed for
maximal variety. It was, for Winnicott, not a question of
what was real about human beings – which would presup-
pose a known essence – but of what, for each person, 'gives
the feeling of real'. This could only be found by each person
for himself.

The experience of aliveness, Winnicott had discovered,
could not be taken for granted. There were people who had
experienced such severe failure of the early holding environment that they felt they had not started to exist. Their lives
were characterized by a sense of futility born of compliance.
Psychoanalysis became, for these people, the provision of
an environment in which, Winnicott writes, 'the patient

will find his or her own self, and will be able to exist and to feel real. Feeling real is more than existing; it is finding a way to exist as oneself, and to relate to objects as oneself, and to have a self into which to retreat for relaxation.'[3] Winnicott assumes that everyone 'has' a self that, like a plant, depends for its realization on a nurturing environment. But to begin with, 'the self of the infant . . . is only potential'.[4] It is gradually constituted through recognition by the mother of the infant's spontaneous gestures, through being reliably seen by her; and it is consolidated through aggression, the mother's survival – meaning her non-retaliation – of the infant and child's destructiveness. In three important papers that can be usefully read as a series – 'The Mirror-Role of Mother and Family in Child Development' (1967),[5] 'The Use of an Object and Relating through Identifications' (1969),[6] and 'Ego Distortion in Terms of True and False Self' (1960)[7] – Winnicott provides a final statement of his developmental theory.

As we have seen, each of Winnicott's contributions to psychoanalytic theory came out of his always evolving sense of what mothers did for their infants. In 'The Mirror-Role' Winnicott suggests that 'the precursor of the mirror is the mother's face' and that the 'mother's role [is] of giving back to the baby the baby's own self'. When the infant looks at the mother's face he can see himself, how he feels, reflected back in her expression. If she is preoccupied by something else, when he looks at her he will only see how *she* feels. He will not be able to get 'something of [himself] back from the environment'. He can only discover what he feels by seeing it reflected back. If the infant is seen in a way that makes him feel he exists, in a way that confirms him, he is free to go on looking.

The mother's face is an essential feature in the process Winnicott describes of an object being presented 'in such a way that the baby's legitimate experience of omnipotence is not violated'. If the object is unable to respond to the infant's gesture of personal need 'the central self suffers insult'. If the mother is unable to fit in with her baby at the beginning, he will be unable to recognize himself in her distracted response. By direct analogy psychoanalysis, Winnicott proposes, 'is a complex derivative of the face that reflects what is there to be seen'. Like the mother's long-term tending of her infant and child, psychoanalysis is a 'giving the patient back what the patient brings'.

The French analyst Lacan had proposed, in a seminal paper to which Winnicott refers, 'Le Stade du miroir' (1949),[8] that when the child looked in the mirror he saw a unified image of his own disarray. Though he experienced himself as all over the place, in bits and pieces, he observed himself collected into an image. This disparity – this formative misrecognition – offered the child the lure of a spurious image of completeness that would, in actuality, forever seduce and elude him. The mirror, Lacan suggested, was deeply misleading, it gave the child a false promise. But for Winnicott what the child saw in the mirror was determined by his experience of the mother's face. If his mother is sufficiently responsive the child experiences himself being seen 'for what he in fact [is] at any moment'. A sense of misrecognition, or a feeling of conflict in the child, Winnicott sees, predictably perhaps, as the consequence of a failure of the maternal provision. Mirrors, like mothers before them, could be usefully looked into, because they were potentially, in the fullest sense, reflective. Just like Winnicott's good-enough mother, they could be reliable and accurate in their acknowledgement.

But the child can only begin looking by first seeing himself, 'being seen is at the basis of creative looking'. Perception – looking at things – is an addition to, but must never be separated from, apperception – seeing oneself. The child with an unresponsive mother – the mother whose face is frozen by a depressed mood – is forced to perceive, to read the mood at the cost of his own feelings being recognized. This perception that pre-empts apperception is an early form of compliance; unable to get 'the mirror to notice and approve' the child, in the simple reversal I have described, is compelled to see only what the mother feels. And he has no way of knowing what, if anything, he has contributed to her mood.

There is, Winnicott suggests, a 'historical process (in the individual) which depends on being seen:

> When I look I am seen, so I exist.
> I can now afford to look and see.
> I now look creatively and what I apperceive I also perceive.
> In fact I take care not to see what is not there to be seen (unless I am tired).'[9]

Not to be seen by the mother, at least at the moment of the spontaneous gesture, is not to exist. In Winnicott's account, being seen by the mother is being recognized for who one is, and what the infant is, is what he feels. The infant cannot risk looking, if looking draws a blank; he must get something of himself back from what he looks at. This makes the mother of infancy the arbiter of the infant's truth. Her responsive recognition – not, for example, a conflict of recognitions between them – makes up his sense of himself. The mother is the constitutive witness of the True Self. If she violates the infant's initial omnipotence – forcing him to see her – she 'insults' the infant's self and drives it into hiding. Everything hinges on the changeover from mother as a subjective object to an object objectively perceived; from seeing himself through the other, to seeing the other. It is a process in which the infant, not the mother, must take the lead. Forcing the pace can only be managed by the infant through compliance.

But if the infant feels real, at the very beginning, through the mother's reflective recognition, how does this develop into contact with, and perception of, real other objects? Winnicott describes this process – 'the most difficult thing, perhaps, in human development' – as the changeover from relating to objects to use of objects. 'From relating to usage' is his description of the shift from the infant's experience of a subjective object to one objectively perceived and outside omnipotent control. To be used, in Winnicott's sense, the object must be real; and the capacity to use objects is not an automatic development but depends, absolutely, on a facilitating object.

In 'The Use of an Object' Winnicott gives a lucid account of this process, from relating to usage, that necessitates a 'statement of the positive value of destructiveness'. And in this simple statement Winnicott makes his final, and in some ways decisive, revision of the work of Freud and Klein. If, in Winnicott's terms, the self is first made real through recognition, the object is first made real through aggressive destruction; and this, of course, makes experience of the object feel real to the self. The object, Winnicott says, is placed outside omnipotent control by being destroyed while, in fact, surviving the destruction. Winnicott offers his own mock-Punch-and-Judy dialogue to illustrate his point:

> The subject says to the object: 'I destroyed you', and the object is there to receive the communication. From now on the subject says: 'Hullo object!' 'I destroyed you.' 'I love you. You have value for me because of your survival of my destruction of you. While I am loving you I am all the time destroying you in (unconscious) *fantasy*.'[10]

It is the backdrop of destruction – in fantasy – that keeps the object real, and so available for use. But the object must be there to receive the communication. If the object will not allow itself to be destroyed, and does not retaliate: if it survives the full blast of the subject's destructiveness, then, and only then, can the subject conceive of the object as beyond his power and therefore fully real. The self and the other have to collaborate; their reality for each other is mutually constituted. 'It is the destruction of the object', Winnicott writes, emphasizing the point, 'that places the object outside of the area of the subject's omnipotent control. In these ways the object develops its own autonomy and life and (if it survives) contributes in to the subject, according to its own properties.'[11] Through the infant's and child's cumulative experience of destruction withstood – of an object resilient (non-rejecting) in the way the hostels for the evacuated children had to be resilient – 'a world of shared reality is created', Winnicott writes, 'which the subject can use and which can feed back other-than-me substance.' Patients deprived of this crucial early experience will need analysis to enable them to develop a capacity to use objects. Then, Winnicott writes, 'the essential feature is the analyst's survival and the intactness of the psychoanalytic technique.'

But this developmental process from relating to usage is a significant modification of psychoanalytic theory. In Freud or, as Winnicott writes more covertly, 'orthodox theory', the object is destroyed *because* it is beyond omnipotent control, its independent reality frustrates. For Winnicott it is the 'destructive drive that creates the quality of external-ity'; and it is the externality, the separate reality of the object, that makes it available for satisfaction. It is destruc-tiveness, paradoxically, that creates reality, not reality that creates destructiveness. So for Winnicott, Klein's concept of the depressive position now seemed more like a protection-racket, a sophisticated version of being nice to mother. In Winnicott's view the object was not reconstituted by the

132

subject's reparation – as Klein believed – but constituted by its own survival.

The mother – as we have seen, that original Winnicottian analyst – must recognize and reflect back what the infant initiates, and must be resilient in a non-retaliatory way when the infant seeks the recognition inherent in destructiveness. It is part of Winnicott's demand on the mother that she be robust; if she is in any way rejecting, the infant has to comply with her response. It is the strategies of compliance that Winnicott calls the False Self Organization. Because of this primary and enforced attentiveness to the needs of the mother, the False Self, he writes, always 'lacks something, and that something is the *essential element of creative originality*'.[12] The creative originality that Winnicott considered to be an innate characteristic of infancy, realized through maternal care, could be muffled or felt to be lost.

In 'The True and False Self' Winnicott links 'the idea of a True Self with the spontaneous gesture'; this, he believes, is the beginning of a feeling of existing and feeling real, and depends upon what he refers to elsewhere as 'a basic ration of the experience of omnipotence'.[13] 'The protest against being forced into a false existence', the premature abrogation of omnipotence, 'can be detected', he writes, 'from the earliest stages'.[14] There is, he implies, an innate authenticity. But if the infant is unable to 'start by existing not by reacting' then he will have to develop a False Self as a measure of protection, 'a defence against that which is unthinkable, the exploitation of the True Self, which would result in annihilation'. The False Self, an 'idea which our patients give us', has three functions: it attends, within severe limitations, to the mother; it hides and protects the True Self by complying with environmental demands; and it is also a 'caretaker' (another 'patient's word'), like a nurse looking after a child, taking over the caring function of the environment that has failed. It is a primitive form of self-sufficiency in the absence of nurture. It begins to emerge, in its severest form, in infancy:

> The good-enough mother meets the omnipotence of the infant and to some extent makes sense of it. She does this repeatedly. A True Self begins to have life, through the strength given to the infant's weak ego ·by the mother's implementation of the infant's omnipotent expressions.
>
> The mother who is not good-enough is not able to implement the infant's omnipotence, and so she repeatedly fails to meet the infant's gesture; instead she substitutes her own gesture which is to be given sense by the compliance of the infant. This compliance on the part of the infant is the earliest stage of the False Self, and belongs to the mother's inability to sense her infant's needs.[15]

The mother implements in the sense of fulfilling the infant's gesture by her response. If she is unable to respond to him through identification he must compulsively comply in order to survive. The False Self organization, at its most extreme, 'results in a feeling unreal or a sense of futility'. But there are, Winnicott makes clear, 'degrees' of False Self, and these can be summarized, beginning with the most severe case, as follows:

1. The False Self replaces and appears to be the real person, while the True Self is so hidden as to seem absent.

2. The False Self protects the True Self that is 'acknowledged as a potential and is allowed a secret life'.

3. The False Self has a 'main concern' which is the finding and maintaining of conditions, of an environment 'which will make it possible for the True Self to come into its own'. The False Self, 'built on identifications', copies others to protect the True Self from misrecognition.

4. The False Self represents an ordinarily adaptive 'social manner'. It is the healthy compromise of socialized politeness that is seen as such, a 'not wearing the heart on the sleeve'. This both maintains and implicitly acknowledges a more private personal self.

The True Self, by contrast, cannot be said to have degrees. It cannot strictly speaking be defined because it covers what is distinctive and original about each person. It is simply a category for the idiosyncratic. 'There is but little point in formulating a True Self idea,' Winnicott writes, 'except for the purpose of trying to understand the False Self.' In broad outline it can be characterized in the following way:

1. At first it is 'the theoretical position from which comes the spontaneous gesture and the personal idea. The spontaneous gesture is the True Self in action.'
2. The True Self is the source of what is authentic in a person. 'Only the True Self can be creative,' Winnicott insists, 'and only the True Self can feel real.'
3. The True Self is bound up with bodily aliveness. It is 'little more than the summation of sensory-motor aliveness'. In fact it 'comes from the aliveness of the body-tissues and the working of the body-functions, including the heart's action and breathing'.
4. As it is what is original about a person that derives from 'inherited potential', it is 'at the beginning, essentially not reactive to external stimuli, but primary'.
5. The True Self is the body as creative.

Somewhere between the True Self and the False Self Winnicott mentions – as a transitional figure, as it were – the actor as the paradoxical man:

> In regard to actors, there are those who can be themselves and who also can act, whereas there are others who can only act, and who are completely at a loss

when not in a role, and when not being appreciated or applauded (acknowledged as existing).[16]

The distinction is between choosing to act as part of a repertoire of ways of being, and being unable to do anything but act, as a derivative of early compliance. Winnicott even suggests, in a characteristically oblique sentence, that 'it may even be possible for the child to act a special role, that of the True Self *as it would be if it had had existence*'.[17] Is it possible to enact an idea of authenticity, and where would the idea come from if it was possible? Winnicott leaves his most extraordinary (and perhaps fruitful) idea about the Self in italics, but unelaborated.

His late division of the Self into True and False elements could not, despite his disclaimers, be easily linked with Freud's concepts of the Id and the Ego. The True Self was not a 'seething cauldron' of instincts, as Freud had once described the Id; and the Ego, which does bear some comparison with the False Self, could never have been described by Freud as a nurse. Winnicott had built his theory out of the self-descriptions of patients, not out of a special language that was divorced from clinical work; there were inevitably drawbacks to its application. One can imagine, for example, a person describing a part of himself as false because it was unacceptable, but nevertheless truly a part of him. It was, perhaps, misleading to refer to a part of the self that looked after another part as 'false', and an essentially indefinable part as True. And yet through his use of an albeit idiosyncratic ordinary language, Winnicott made the theory of psychoanalysis more accessible to people it was originally intended to help.

But given psychoanalysis had been traditionally conceived of as a treatment in words, what was the relationship of language to this elusive True Self? Could it, like the Unconscious, speak (albeit in disguise), or be spoken to? It was certainly not, like the Unconscious, intrinsically unacceptable. Winnicott, in fact, never confronted the difficulty of relating his True Self concept to Freud's concept of the Unconscious. As he got older he developed his own ideas in virtual disregard of the traditional languages of psychoanalysis. But it was to the role of language in psychoanalytic treatment, and its tenuous relationship with the True Self, that Winnicott turned his attention in the last years of his life.

137

6 The Play of Interpretation

'It is good to love the unknown.'

Charles Lamb

In virtually every paper Winnicott wrote, he says something explicitly about language, though he tends to speak of 'words' rather than the more panoramic idea of Language as a system. And yet all his major contributions to psychoanalysis are based on a theory of infancy. As he points out in a section of his paper 'The Theory of the Parent–Infant Relationship' (1960) entitled The Word Infant: 'Actually the word infant implies "not talking" (infans) and it is not unuseful to think of infancy as the phase prior to word presentation and the use of word symbols.'[1] The double negative that is common in Winnicott's writing may compact a doubt. But whereas for Freud psychoanalysis was essentially a 'talking cure' dependent on two people speaking to each other, for Winnicott the mother–infant relationship, in which communication was relatively non-verbal, had become the paradigm for the analytic process, and this changed the role of interpretation in psychoanalytic treatment. For the neurotic and the psychotic patient, for the child and the adult, interpretation was a sophisticated extension of infant care, albeit a crucial part of the analyst's primary aim in the treatment which was to establish and maintain an environment conducive to growth. The defining characteristic of the analytic setting for Winnicott was not exclusively verbal exchange.

In the work of the British School linguistics was never seen as a complementary discipline to psychoanalysis. Lan-

138

guage, in Winnicott's developmental theory, merely extends the child's capacity for communication and separateness, but is not in itself considered formative of his identity. He makes nothing in his work, for example, of the connection between the child's acquisition of language and his shift from a two-person to a three-person relationship. He believed in the continuity, not the constitutive differences, between 'the vitally important subtle communicating of the infant–mother kind', the child playing and beginning to speak, and the adult talking. And he was blithely dismissive, on occasions, of the distinction between language and other forms of representation. Comparing child and adult analysis, he wrote that 'the difference between the child and the adult is that the child often plays rather than talks. The difference, however, is almost without significance and indeed some adults draw or play.'[2] The difference seems relatively unimportant to Winnicott because there are other forms of representation available for use; talking is only one part of the repertoire. Language is something which, Winnicott believes, is simply 'added' at a later stage to the infant's primary capacity for communication. It is the sociability from the very beginning, that predates language, that Winnicott's work is based on.

The infant does not speak but he survives because he communicates with a receptive object. But Winnicott's use of a pre-linguistic model – the mother–infant relationship – for the treatment with words that is the defining characteristic of psychoanalysis, has problematic implications. The difference that language makes, like the difference the father makes, is never theoretically elaborated by Winnicott. And infancy, which, it is assumed, can be described and spoken of, cannot, of course, speak for itself; it is exempt from one thing language makes possible and that psychoanalysis depends upon, the construction of a personal history. Can that which is experienced pre-reflectively, in

139

the body but without language, be reached through language? There is, Winnicott implies, a language of maternal care, that is not made only of words.

Verbal interpretation in analysis is, for Winnicott, a form of mothering. 'What matters to the patient', he writes – and it is with what matters to the patient that Winnicott is always keen to concern himself –

> is not the accuracy of the interpretation so much as the willingness of the analyst to help, the analyst's capacity to identify with the patient and so to believe in what is needed and to meet the need as soon as the need is indicated verbally or in non-verbal or pre-verbal language.[3]

The act of interpretation, aside from its content, expresses collaborative concern; it comes out of identifying with the patient – being able, to some extent, to imagine what it is like to be that person at that moment – and then the more unexpected consequence of 'believing in' what he needs. Identification here, for Winnicott, like Primary Maternal Preoccupation, implies a commitment. In fact the process of willingness, belief in, and meeting are all suggestive of his almost religious sense of the mother's 'ordinary devotion' to her infant (even though 'ordinary', like 'natural', in Winnicott's writing often expresses a wish). The analyst in Winnicott's account is not only, as Freud wrote, 'disclosing to [the patient] the hidden meaning of the ideas that occur to him',[4] he is using interpretation to signify maternal care. The analytic setting is a medium for personal growth not exclusively the provision of a convincing translation of the unconscious.

If it is 'the innate tendencies towards integration and growth that produce health, not the environmental provision',[5] then, by the same token, 'it is axiomatic', Winnicott writes, 'that the work of the analysis is done by the patient.'[6]

The analyst, like the mother, facilitates by providing opportunity for communication and its recognition. Just as a feed
can be seen as an interpretation of the infant's cry by the
mother, so the analyst's verbal interpretations can be like a
feed for the patient in language. For Winnicott, these are
simple and accurate equivalents on a developmental continuum. In 'The Theory of the Parent–Infant Relationship'
Winnicott describes what is by now a familiar process. At
first, we may remember, it is as though the infant is merged
in with the mother who seems to him to have 'an almost
magical understanding of [his] need'. As they separate out
and there is 'a disentanglement of maternal care from
something which we then call the infant', the mother
notices that the infant no longer expects this magical
understanding. 'The mother seems to know', he writes,
'that the infant has a new capacity, that of giving a signal so
that she can be guided towards meeting the infant's needs.
It could be said that if now she knows too well what the
infant needs, this is magic and forms no basis for an object-
relationship.'[7]

In the merged state the mother is exclusively a subjective
object which precludes the need for anything the infant
could conceive of as a signal. If she 'knows too well', then
from the infant's point of view he is not relating to an
external object. But Winnicott describes this development
from being merged in to being separate and requiring some
kind of language as a natural process given good-enough
mothering. And he assumes that the infant's capacity to
signal is akin to the adult's acquisition of language; language is seen as the sophisticated giving of signals. So
Winnicott can make a direct comparison between the infant
giving a signal to the mother and the patient talking in
analysis. 'It is very important,' he writes, 'except when the
patient is regressed to earliest infancy, that the analyst shall
not know the answers except insofar as the patient gives

141

the clues.'[8] Magical interpretations pre-empt the patient's separateness; he is robbed of a mind of his own. The mother does not give the infant a feed, the infant gives the mother the opportunity to feed him. The clues provided by the patient facilitate the analyst's capacity to interpret. 'It is not so much a question of giving the baby satisfaction,' and the comparison with the analytic situation is implicit, 'as of letting the baby find and come to terms with the object.'[9]

Critical of the 'silent analyst', Winnicott interprets, he says, because 'if I make none the patient gets the impression that I understand everything. In other words, I retain some outside quality by not being quite on the mark – or even by being wrong.'[10] Winnicott is acutely sensitive to the ways in which the analyst, by virtue of the psychoanalytic situation itself, can become a seductive impostor of the omniscient mother. He aims to be an attentive but unimpinging object. Through brief, 'economical' interpretations – 'I never use long sentences unless I am very tired'[11] – he communicates to the patient that he is not a usurping presence. Since in Winnicott's version the mother–infant relationship is defined by its reciprocity – the 'illusion' that makes exchange between them possible, sustained by mutual participation – then the conversation that is psychoanalysis becomes analogous to play. For Winnicott the opposite of play is not work but coercion. This means, of course, that the analyst has to be able to play as well. It is in the overlap, the transitional space between analyst and patient, that communication takes place. Playing stops when one of the participants becomes dogmatic, when the analyst imposes a pattern that is not of a piece with the patient's material. 'Interpretation outside the ripeness of the material', Winnicott writes, 'is indoctrination and produces compliance. A corollary is that resistance arises out of interpretation given outside the area of overlap of the patient's and the analyst's playing together.'[12] There can be no right interpretation that is beyond the patient's recognition. The patient's resistance, in Winnicott's view, is not integral to the psychoanalytic enterprise, as Freud believed, but reflects the analyst's failure to play. The unacceptable interpretation, like a maternal impingement, can only be reacted to by the patient, not taken in and used. 'An interpretation that does not work', Winnicott writes in the Introduction to his *Therapeutic Consultations in Child Psychiatry*, 'always means that I have made the interpretation at the wrong moment or in the wrong way, and I withdraw it unconditionally . . . Dogmatic interpretation leaves the child with only two alternatives, an *acceptance* of what I have said as propaganda, or a *rejection* of the interpretation and of me and of the whole set-up.'[13] Winnicott believes that the child knows what interests him; the interpretation, just like the spatula, cannot be forced into the patient's mouth. It is there to be used, in the way Winnicott described the Transitional Object as being used, not revered, copied, or complied with. And because it is essentially transitional to an unknowable destination, it could never be conclusive. A good interpretation, one could say, is something the patient can entertain in his mind. It is not a password.

Since Winnicott was consistently preoccupied, as we have seen, with the transitional rather than the conclusive in human experience – committed to growth, not the acquiring of convictions – interpretation was always in the service of a developmental process in which knowing and being known had an increasingly equivocal status for him. The final decade of his work is marked by a profound ambivalence about the knowability of the self that is matched by a certain reticence about the value of the analyst as interpreter. For both patient and analyst playing replaced knowing as the aim and the means of analysis. The mother, and her later counterpart, the analyst, could enable but should not, in Winnicott's view, inform or teach. They both were facilitators of an ongoing developmental process which they had not invented and in which the will to comprehensive understanding was redundant. 'There are those who fear to wait and who implant,' Winnicott writes in a distinction that is at the centre of his work, 'just as there are those who wait, and keep ready for presentation the ideas and expectations that the child can use on his arrival at each new developmental stage of integration and capacity for objective consideration.'[14] It is through play that the child begins to include in his personal pattern of preoccupation those things he is ready for, that he finds himself interested in and enjoying. It is in this sense that for Winnicott the capacity to play was integral to the developmental process and not the capacity he rarely mentions but which had defined the psychoanalytic project, the capacity to know oneself. Insight is a word he rarely uses and one that cannot be found in the indexes to his books. Playing is the process of finding through pleasure what interests you, but it is by definition a state of transitional knowing, creative by virtue of being always inconclusive. And, of course, though there is word-play, playing is not exclusively verbal.

II

'Psychoanalysis', he wrote in his last book, *Playing and Reality*, 'has been developed as a highly specialized form of playing in the service of communication with oneself and others.'[15] It is in his later work that communicating with oneself, of which not communicating with anyone else can be a part, became one of Winnicott's central concerns. It provides the subject of his greatest paper, 'Communicating and Not Communicating Leading to a Study of Certain Opposites' (1963).[16] His continued study, over forty years, of dependency and the mother–infant relationship had led him to a belief in 'the permanent isolation of the individual'. The paradox that he had begun to formulate was that the infant – like the adolescent about whom he could only write authoritatively in the last decade of his life – was an isolate who needed the object, above all, to protect the privacy of this isolation. It was maternal nurture that kept the essential privacy of the developmental process alive. 'We can understand', he writes, 'the hatred people have of psychoanalysis which has penetrated a long way into the human personality, and which provides a threat to the human individual in his need to be secretly isolated.'[17] It is a striking use of one of Winnicott's favoured ideas, the idea of provision. This paper can be seen, I think, as, among the other things, Winnicott's belated attempt to understand his own resistance to psychoanalysis, which involved him in defining the self as essentially secret.

Adolescents, he suggests, 'eschew psychoanalytic treatment, though they are interested in psychoanalytic theories' because their 'preservation of personal isolation is part of the search for identity, and for the establishment of a personal technique for communicating which does not lead to violation of the central self'.[18] Violation of the central self refers to the self-betrayal born of compliance; identity is bound up for Winnicott with this search for a personal way of communicating that is not compromised by concession to the object. In 'Morals and Education' (1963) he explicitly values 'those who do not copy and comply, but who genuinely grow to a way of personal expression'.[19] Because he was fearful of his own ventriloquism, of speaking someone else's language – which is to some extent what language always is – he tended to idolize the individual voice as a way of protecting its possibility. His work was increasingly the attempt to understand what precluded the emergence of the individual voice.

The 'danger' of psychoanalysis, he believed, could be

located at that specific developmental point which we have looked at, and which he keeps referring to in his later writing: the moment when the analyst in the transference changes over from being a subjective object to an object objectively perceived. It is at such moments that the patient's experience of omnipotence can be violated, and the analyst impinges:

> here there is danger if the analyst interprets instead of waiting for the patient to creatively discover . . . If we wait we become objectively perceived in the patient's own time, but if we fail to behave in a way that is facilitating the patient's analytic process (which is the equivalent of the infant's and the child's maturational process) we suddenly become not-me for the patient, and then we know too much, and we are dangerous because we are too nearly in communication with the central still and silent spot of the patient's ego-organization.[20]

The interpretation, like the object, is only good to the patient if it is felt to be created by him: and yet, Winnicott writes, 'the object must be found in order to be created. This has to be accepted as a paradox.' Analyst and patient, like mother and infant, work in that intermediate area of illusion which is always vulnerable to pre-emptive intrusion. But in this paper Winnicott implies that language, in the form of an accurate interpretation for which the patient is not ready, can reach into his innermost being, evoke his most primitive defences. It suddenly acquires an unexpected potency. 'Rape and being eaten by cannibals,' Winnicott writes, 'these are mere bagatelles as compared with the violation of the self's core, the alteration of the self's central elements by communication seeping through the defences.'[21] Language, in this context, is potentially a terrifying maternal object. In writing this paper, in fact, Winnicott says that he found himself 'staking a claim, to my surprise, to the right not to communicate. This was a protest from the core of me to the frightening fantasy of being infinitely exploited . . . the fantasy of being found.'[22] For Winnicott surprise authenticates: he suggests there is a primitive terror in the form of a simple equation – to be found means to be exploited. And he takes it for granted here that a person can be found in language. The overinterpretative analyst becomes the tyrannical mother, and language is integral to her power. So Winnicott uses this paper to distinguish between 'pathological withdrawal and healthy central self-communication': the child's need to escape into himself away from the intrusive mother, from the mother having facilitated in her infant satisfying contact with himself. The origin of this satisfying self-communion he describes in a complementary paper, 'The Capacity to be Alone' (1958),[23] as the child being contentedly alone in the presence of his mother. The person's relationship with himself begins to take centre-stage in Winnicott's theory-making.

Winnicott describes a repertoire of three 'forms' of communication. 'In the best possible circumstances', he writes,

> growth takes place and the child now possesses three lines of communication: communication that is *for ever silent*, communication that is *explicit*, indirect and pleasurable, and this third or *intermediate* form of communication that slides out of playing into cultural experience of every kind.[24]

The first kind of communication, Winnicott suggests, in a puzzling double negative, is 'not non-verbal; it is, like the music of the spheres, absolutely personal. It belongs to being alive.'[25] Winnicott offers an elusive paradox here to deal with the possible contradiction of the idea of a private language (how does one learn it, and where does it come from if not from outside?). Although he does not say so, the dream, perhaps, provides the most compelling example of what he is talking about. But the music of the spheres – which, like the dream, one does not hear – was produced, Pythagoras said, by the essentially harmonious movement of the spheres. This non-conflictual analogy is used to illustrate Winnicott's favoured form of communication, linked for him with feeling real.

The second form of communication Winnicott associates with verbal language. By being what he calls indirect but explicit – a shrewd association of ideas about language – language protects the separateness, the isolation of the self. He refers to children becoming 'masters of various techniques for indirect communication',[26] as though these techniques were like Transitional Objects, not complied with but used. There is no sense here, it should be noted, of language being subtler than the intentions of its users. And Winnicott never makes clear to what extent it is through the acquisition of language that the mother becomes an object objectively perceived, or whether language is acquired as a consequence of this process. Certainly, in this account, verbal language, like other Transitional Phenomena, joins by separating and separates by joining the mother and her developing child. The third, intermediate form of communication, Winnicott says, is 'a most valuable compromise' between the other two kinds, a compromise between language and silence.

But for Winnicott the main point of his paper is that communication with an external object involves a compromising concession on the part of the self. The object always, to some degree, invites compliance. 'At the core of the individual', Winnicott writes, 'there is no communication with the not-me world either way.'[27] There is, however, a contradiction he cannot resolve. He proposes an absolute insulation at the core of the self and then also says that the problem for the individual is how to stay isolated without being insulated. It is as though at the end of his life the issue he had always struggled with, of separation and connectedness, had changed from being an inter-psychic problem between mother and child, to being an intra-psychic problem about a person's relationship with the core of himself. And it is worth noting once again that Winnicott takes his language for an 'essential' self from a simpler form of organic life: the core is the central casing of a fruit that contains the seeds.

Winnicott suggests in this paper that ordinary human development involves a benign version of the splitting of the personality that one finds in severe psychopathology. 'The traumatic experiences that lead to the organization of primitive defences belong', he writes, 'to the threat to the isolated core, the threat of its being found, altered, communicated with. The defence consists in the further hiding of the secret self.'[28] Each psychoanalytic theorist, it could be said, organizes his or her theory around what might be called a core catastrophe; for Freud it was castration, for Klein, the triumph of the Death instinct, and for Winnicott it was the annihilation of the core self by intrusion, a failure of the holding environment. To understand the hide-and-seek of the self, Winnicott examines what he calls the two opposites of communication. One is a 'simple not-communicating', and the other a 'not-communicating that is active or reactive'. Simple not-communicating is like a period of rest after which, and in one's own time, one goes back to it. It is the second one, in which health and pathology overlap, that preoccupies Winnicott. If the maternal provision fails – and to some extent it must, by definition, fail – then 'in the matter of object-relating the infant has developed a split'.[29] With one half of the split he relates to the available object and develops a false, compliant self to do so, and with the other half he relates to a subjective object, one of his own invention. This involves 'active non-communication

149

with that which is objectively perceived by the infant'. Despite the impoverishment that the split creates – the absence of modification or enrichment from outside – this communication with subjective objects 'carries', Winnicott says, 'all the sense of real'.[30] In what he calls the 'slighter illnesses', the neuroses of everyday life, there is always, Winnicott says, some active non-communication 'because of the fact that communication so easily becomes linked with some degree of false or compliant object-relating; silent or secret communication with subjective objects, carrying a sense of real, must periodically take over to restore the balance.'[31] There is, Winnicott makes clear, a strain built into object-relating. But secrecy, we should note, is different from silence; a secret can be found out, silence is, so to speak, invisible. They are both words Winnicott uses when writing about the True Self.

In the healthy person, Winnicott writes, there is the equivalent – what he refers to enigmatically as 'something that corresponds to' – 'the state of the split person in whom one part of the split communicates silently with subjective objects. There is room for the idea that significant relating and communicating is silent.' There is, he insists, and it is rather like an article of faith, 'the healthy use of non-communication in the establishment of the feeling of real'.[32] The feeling of real that for Winnicott was synonymous with health and development was not constituted linguistically, nor exclusively in relation to the other, though self-communion of the kind he describes is only possible through the experience of good-enough early care that protects the possibility of the self. So for Winnicott what might be called the non-verbal silences in analytic treatment are as potentially fertile as verbal exchange: they signify the secret metabolism of the self. So Freud's work, built on by Winnicott, makes a new kind of silence possible. Indeed, one of the aims of analysis may be to facilitate such silences in the patient.

Winnicott defines the self in this paper as isolated, secret and silent. It can only be understood in terms of a profound ambivalence about the value of communicating with external objects. 'The individual knows', he writes, 'that [the true self] must never be communicated with or be influenced by external reality',[33] but it is as though communication is equivalent to influence and that influence is malign (one of the early precursors of this paper is entitled 'On Influencing and Being Influenced', 1941[34]). 'Although healthy persons communicate and enjoy communicating, the other fact is equally true', he writes, 'that *each individual is an isolate, permanently non-communicating, permanently unknown, in fact unfound.*'[35] This is unusually insistent for Winnicott. It is, on the one hand, a passionate commitment to the privacy of the self. But on the other hand it may also be true that if the analyst offers himself up as primarily a maternal object, his need for privacy, his fears about being exploited, will eventually reassert themselves.

Once again it is the figure of the artist who embodies the drive for authenticity that is for Winnicott exemplary for that integrity of being he values above all else. 'In the artist of all kinds', he writes, 'one can detect an inherent dilemma, which belongs to the co-existence of two trends, the urgent need to communicate and the still more urgent need not to be found. This might account for the fact that we cannot conceive of an artist's coming to the end of the task that occupies his whole nature.'[36] Development is primarily comparable for Winnicott to the project of the artist whose most urgent need, he now believed in the last years of his life, is not to be found. For Freud, towards the end of his life, there was the conflict between the two instincts of Life and Death, Eros and Thanatos. For Winnicott there was the conflict between two trends, to communicate and to hide.

151

The self is, by definition, elusive, the player of hide and seek.[37]

In a review of Jung's autobiography, *Memories, Dreams, Reflections*, one of the most revealing pieces Winnicott ever wrote, he suggested:

> If I want to say that Jung was mad, and that he recovered, I am doing nothing worse than I would do in saying of myself that I was sane and through analysis and self-analysis I achieved some measure of insanity. Freud's flight to sanity could be something we psycho-analysts are trying to recover from, just as Jungians are trying to recover from Jung's 'divided self', and from the way he himself dealt with it.[38]

Placing himself in the tradition, Winnicott offers us a choice: sanity, a divided self, or the achievement of 'some measure of insanity'. It is a characteristically paradoxical phrase. If there could be Winnicottians they would have to recover from Winnicott's flight into infancy, his flight from the erotic. But his measure of insanity is, I think, an inspiration.

CHRONOLOGY

1896   Born on 7 April in Plymouth of Methodist parents, the youngest of three children (his sisters were Violet, b.1890, and Cathleen, b.1891). His father, John Frederick Winnicott, was a corsetry merchant, born in 1855, a year before Freud.

1910   Attends Leys School in Cambridge, specializing in sciences.

1916   Goes to Jesus College, Cambridge, to read medicine.

1917   In November joins the Navy until the end of the war.

1918   Goes to Bart's Hospital in London to study medicine.

1919   First reads Freud in Brill's translation of *The Interpretation of Dreams*.

1920   Begins to specialize in paediatrics.

1923   Appointed as consultant in children's medicine at Paddington Green Children's Hospital and Queen's Hospital, Hackney. Marries Alice Taylor, a potter, and begins his analysis with James Strachey, which will finish in 1933.

1924   Begins private practice in Harley Street. His father is knighted.

1925   His mother dies. Melanie Klein lectures in London to the British Society.

1926   Klein moves to London.

1931   Publishes his first book, *Clinical Notes on Disorders of Childhood*.

1933–8   In analysis with Joan Rivière.

1935   Reads his paper 'The Manic Defence' for membership to the British Psychoanalytical Society.

1940   Appointed Psychiatric Consultant to the Government Evacuation Scheme in the County of Oxford; does radio broadcasts for mothers during the war.

1944   Appointed Fellow of the Royal College of Physicians.

1948   On 31 December his father dies; he has his first coronary.

1949   Divorced from his wife.

1951   Marries Clare Britton.

1956–9 President of the British Psychoanalytical Society.

1957   Publishes collections of broadcast talks and papers to lay audiences: *The Child and the Family: First Relationships* and *The Child and the Outside World: Studies in Developing Relationships*.

1958   Publishes his first book of psychoanalytic papers, *Collected Papers: Through Paediatrics to Psycho-Analysis*.

1964   Publishes *The Child, the Family, and the Outside World* (a selection from his two books published in 1957), and *The Family and Individual Development*.

1965   Publishes his second volume of collected papers, *The Maturational Processes and the Facilitating Environment: Studies in the Theory of Emotional Development*.

1965–8 President again of the British Psychoanalytical Society.

1968   Awarded the James Spence Medal for Paediatrics; has a serious heart attack in New York.

1971   Dies in London on 25 January. *Playing and Reality* published, followed by *Therapeutic Consultations in Child Psychiatry*.

NOTES

Introduction

1. Quoted in Davis and Wallbridge 1983, p.24.
2. 'Transitional Objects and Transitional Phenomena' (1951), Winnicott 1971a, p.26.
3. 'Paediatrics and Psychiatry' (1948), Winnicott 1958, p.161.
4. 'Counter-Transference' (1960), Winnicott 1965, p.158.
5. 'Communicating and Not Communicating' (1963), Winnicott 1965, p.187. In Winnicott 1988, p.52, Winnicott states that 'out of the material of the imaginative elaboration of body functioning (which itself depends upon the capacity and healthy functioning of one organ: the brain) the psyche is forged', and that the Soul is 'a property of the psyche'. Leaving aside the ambiguity of 'forged', in this description the Soul is no longer the kind of personal essence suggested by Winnicott's concept of the True Self. It is derivative and constructed rather than given. The religious vocabulary that lurks in Winnicott's psychoanalytic writing often leads him into revealing kinds of confusion. For an interesting account of the relationship between the idea of the Soul and the idea of originality that sheds light, by implication, on many of Winnicott's concerns, see *Originality and Imagination* by Thomas McFarland (Baltimore and London: Johns Hopkins University Press, 1985).
6. 'Residential Management as Treatment for Difficult Children' (written with Clare Britton, 1947), Winnicott 1984, p.58.
7. 'The Contribution of Psycho-Analysis to Midwifery' (1957), Winnicott 1964b, p.110.
8. 'The Family and Emotional Maturity' (1960), Winnicott 1964b, p.94.
9. 'Further Thoughts on Babies as Persons' (1947), Winnicott 1964a, p.88.
10. For a discussion of this central issue in psychoanalytic theory see *Pleasure and Being: Hedonism from a Psycho-Analytic Point of View* by Moustafa Safouan, trans. by Martin Thom (London: Macmillan, 1983).
11. 'The Location of Cultural Experience' (1967), Winnicott 1971a, p.116.
12. Idem.
13. This and related issues are clarified in *War in the Nursery: Theories of the Child and Mother* by Denise Riley (London: Virago, 1983).
14. 'Cure' (1970), Winnicott 1987a, pp.114–15.

15. Introduction, Winnicott 1971b, p.2.
16. Ibid. See 'Living Creatively' (1970), p.53, and 'The Pill and the Moon' (1969), p.197, both in Winnicott 1987a, for further references to surprise. For an Emersonian parallel see Emerson's essay 'Experience' in *Essays* by Ralph Waldo Emerson, edited by Sherman Paul (London: Dent, Everyman, 1906), pp.241–2.
17. 'Cure', op. cit., p.117.
18. 'Primitive Emotional Development' (1945), Winnicott 1958, p.150.
19. 'Paediatrics and Childhood Neurosis' (1956), Winnicott 1958, pp.318–19.
20. 'Mirror-Role of Mother and Family in Child Development' (1967), Winnicott 1971a, p.138.
21. 'Cure', op. cit., p.112.
22. 'The Aims of Psycho-Analytical Treatment' (1962), Winnicott 1965, p.167.
23. 'Playing: a Theoretical Statement' (1971), Winnicott 1971a, p.65.
24. 'The Use of an Object and Relating through Identifications' (1969), Winnicott 1971a, p.108.
25. Greenberg and Mitchell 1983, p.189.
26. 'Playing', op. cit., p.44.
27. 'Primitive Emotional Development', op. cit., p.145.
28. See *The New Ego: Pitfalls in Current Thinking about Patients in Psychoanalysis* by Nathan Leites (New York: Science House, 1971) for a discussion of the notion of 'adopting' that is akin to 'borrowing' as a necessary but mislaid term in psychoanalysis. It is not clear, for example, whether one could conceive of a Transitional Object as something borrowed or adopted from somewhere.
29. Winnicott 1971a, pp.101–12.

1. *What We Call the Beginning*

1. For this and all other autobiographical material in this chapter, unless otherwise stated, see 'D. W. Winnicott: a Reflection' by Clare Winnicott in Grolnick *et al.* 1978.
2. 'Fear of Breakdown', *International Review of Psycho-Analysis*, 1, 1973.
3. Ibid.
4. 'The Location of Cultural Experience' (1967), Winnicott 1971a, p.115.
5. 'Growth and Development in Immaturity' (1950), Winnicott 1964b, p.21.
6. From the Preface to *Forty-Four Sermons* by John Wesley (London, 1746).
7. 'Transitional Objects and Transitional Phenomena' (1951), Winnicott 1958, p.231. Winnicott reiterates at the end of this paper that, 'Should

an adult make claims on us for our acceptance of the objectivity of his subjective phenomena we discern or diagnose madness' (p.241). *Playing and Reality* (in which it was reprinted) can be seen as, among other things, a critique of states of conviction.

8. Introduction by Masud Khan to Winnicott 1958, p.xxii.
9. Unpublished.
10. Introduction by Masud Khan to Winnicott 1986, p.1.
11. 'The Location of Cultural Experience', op. cit., p.121.
12. 'The Capacity to be Alone' (1958), Winnicott 1965, pp.29–36.
13. James Britton: personal communication.
14. 'Children Learning' (1968), Winnicott 1987a, pp.142–9.
15. 'The Effect of Psychotic Parents' (1959), Winnicott 1964b, p.75.
16. In the Winnicott Archive, New York Hospital-Cornell Medical Center.
17. 'Coronary Thrombosis', unpublished talk given in 1957 to the Society for Psychosomatic Research, University College London. Quoted in Davis and Wallbridge 1983, p.25.
18. 'The Pill and the Moon' (1969), Winnicott 1987a, p.205.
19. 'Obituary: Donald Winnicott' by J. P. M. Tizard, *International Journal of Psycho-Analysis*, vol. 52, part 3: 1971.
20. Letter dated 15 November 1919, in Winnicott 1987b, p.2.
21. 'Growth and Development in Immaturity' (1950), Winnicott 1964b, p.21. See Winnicott 1988, p.36, for further comment on the anxiety – or rather, the depression – of influence Winnicott experienced in relation to Freud. 'Almost every aspect of relationships between whole persons', he writes, 'was touched on by Freud himself, and in fact it is very difficult now to contribute except by fresh statement of what is accepted.' It was, of course, the individual's developmental struggle to achieve relationships between whole persons that distinguished Winnicott's contribution to psychoanalysis.
22. 'Training for Child Psychiatry' (1963), Winnicott 1965, p.199. See 'Classification' (1959–64), Winnicott 1965, pp.124–39, which includes the statement that, 'The psycho-analyst . . . can be looked upon as a specialist in history-taking. It is true that this history-taking is a very involved process. A psycho-analytic case description is a series of case histories, a presentation of different versions of the same case, the versions being arranged in layers each of which represents a stage of revelation' (p.132).
23. See Grosskurth 1987 for the significance of this fact in her life.
24. *International Journal of Psycho-Analysis*, 50, p.129: 1969.
25. Strachey's seminal paper was entitled 'The Nature of the Therapeutic Action of Psycho-Analysis', *International Journal of Psycho-Analysis*, 15: 1934.
26. In the Winnicott Archive, New York Hospital-Cornell Medical

Center: the letters are to Ian Roger and dated 28 May 1969 and 3 June 1969 respectively.

2. History-taking

1. Freud's daughter Anna, however, did attend the Congress. 'According to her telegraphic reports', Freud wrote to Lou Andreas-Salomé, 'Anna is having rather a hard time in Oxford . . . As to the accommodation, she writes, as one might expect: "More tradition than comfort." I expect you know that the English, having created the notion of comfort, then refused to have anything more to do with it.' *Sigmund Freud and Lou Andreas-Salomé: Letters*, edited by Ernst Pfeiffer, trans. by William and Elaine Robson-Scott (London: The Hogarth Press and The Institute of Psycho-Analysis, 1972), p.182.
2. 'The Location of Cultural Experience' (1967), Winnicott 1971a, p.117.
3. 'The Becoming of a Psycho-Analyst' (1972), Khan 1974, p.114.
4. Meisel and Kendrick 1986, p.39.
5. 'An Examination of the Klein System of Child Psychology', *Psycho-Analytic Study of the Child*, vol.1 (London: Imago Publishing Company, 1945).
6. Quoted in Grosskurth 1987, p.167.
7. 'A Personal View of the Kleinian Contribution' (1962), Winnicott 1965, p.172.
8. Idem.
9. Ibid., p.173.
10. Ibid., pp.173–4.
11. 'The Aims of Psycho-Analytical Treatment' (1962), Winnicott 1965, p.166.
12. See Grolnick 1978 and Green 1986 for discussion of Winnicott's interest in paradox; and also *Between Existentialism and Marxism* by Jean-Paul Sartre (London: Verso, 1983), p.38, for what psychoanalysis loses when it relinquishes the notion of contradiction. There is clearly a link to be made between Winnicott's preoccupation with paradox and the absence of a third sex.
13. 'Classification' (1959–64), Winnicott 1965, p.126.
14. 'A Personal View of the Kleinian Contribution', op. cit., p.174.
15. 'Classification', op. cit., p.126.
16. 'A Personal View', op. cit., pp.176–7.
17. 'A Note on Normality and Anxiety' (1931), Winnicott 1958, p.20.
18. 'Short Communication on Enuresis', *St Bartholomew's Hospital Journal*, April 1930.
19. *Proceedings of the Royal Society of Medicine 1930–39*, no.2.
20. 'Mental Hygiene in the Pre-School Child' (unpublished, 1930s).

21. 'Skin Changes in Relation to Emotional Disorder', *St John's Hospital Dermatological Society Report*, 1938.
22. Introduction, Winnicott 1971a, p.xiv.
23. 'Skin Changes', op. cit.
24. 'A Note on Normality and Anxiety', op. cit., p.5.
25. 'Skin Changes', op. cit.
26. 'Fidgetiness' (1931), Winnicott 1958, p.23.
27. 'What Do We Mean by a Normal Child?' (1946), Winnicott 1957a, p.103.
28. Idem.
29. Idem.
30. 'Shyness and Nervous Disorders in Children' (1938), Winnicott 1964a, p.211.
31. 'String: a Technique of Communication' (1960), Winnicott 1965, pp.153–7.
32. 'Shyness', op. cit., p.212.
33. 'A Note on Normality', op. cit., pp.19–20.
34. 'The Only Child' (1945), Winnicott 1964b, p.110.
35. 'Shyness', op. cit., p.212.
36. 'A Note on Normality', op. cit., pp.9–11.
37. *Standard Edition*, vol. XII, p.118.
38. 'The Use of an Object' (1969), Winnicott 1971a, p.102.
39. 'Skin Changes', op. cit.
40. See the conclusion to 'Paediatrics and Childhood Neurosis' (1956), Winnicott 1958, p.321, where Winnicott suggests that 'There must be those who dislike psychoanalysis, because of the fact it studies human nature objectively; it invades the realms where previously belief, intuition, and empathy held sway.' There is an intimation here of Winnicott's growing awareness that psychoanalysis itself was potentially intrusive; and he was, of course, to defend in his later work certain kinds of belief, intuition and empathy.
41. 'The Return of the Evacuated Child' (1945), Winnicott 1984, p.44.
42. 'The Location of Cultural Experience', op. cit., p.117.
43. 'The Manic Defence' (1935), Winnicott 1958, pp.129–44.
44. In *Love, Guilt and Reparation* by Melanie Klein (London: The Hogarth Press and The Insitute of Psycho-Analysis, 1975), pp.262–89.
45. Ibid.
46. Ibid.
47. Hanna Segal, *Klein* (London: Fontana Modern Masters, 1979), p.81.
48. 'The Manic Defence', op. cit., pp.143–4.
49. Ibid., p.129.
50. Ibid., p.130.
51. Idem.
52. See 'Dreaming, Fantasying, and Living' (1971), Winnicott 1971a,

pp.31–43. In Freud's important paper 'Formulations on the Two Principles of Mental Functioning' (1911), *Standard Edition* vol. XII, pp.213–26, Freud suggests that 'With the introduction of the reality principle one species of thought-activity was split off; it was kept free from reality-testing and remained subordinated to the pleasure-principle alone. This activity is phantasying, which begins already in children's play, and later, continued as day-dreaming, abandons dependence on real objects.' Winnicott characteristically takes over Freud's word without acknowledgement, changes the spelling in a significant way, and uses it to describe something related to but notably different from Freud's sense. For Freud, phantasying is the inevitable consequence of the reality principle, and provides a compensatory inner area of freedom. In Winnicott's work fantasying 'remains an isolated phenomenon, absorbing energy but not contributing-in either to dreaming or to living.' It is a stultifying solution to an early failure of mutuality with the environment, a mental activity in which nothing happens.

53. *Standard Edition*, vol. IX, p.192.
54. 'The Manic Defence', op. cit., p.131.
55. 'Reparation in Respect of Mother's Organized Defence against Depression' (1948), Winnicott 1958, p.94.
56. Little 1985.

3. War-time

1. Letter to the *British Medical Journal* (16 December 1939), Winnicott 1984, p.14.
2. 'The Problem of Homeless Children', by D. W. Winnicott and C. Britton, *Children's Communities Monograph No. 1*, 1944. This important article was also published in *The New Era in Home and School*, 25.
3. One could say, for example, that the patient recreates (tries to repeat) in the transference ways of being understood, or forms of understanding, from the past.
4. 'Children in the War' (1940), Winnicott 1984, p.28.
5. 'The Deprived Mother' (1939), Winnicott 1984, p.33.
6. 'Residential Management as Treatment for Difficult Children' (written with C. Britton, 1947), Winnicott 1984, p.60.
7. Ibid., p.55.
8. 'Children in the War', op. cit., p.27.
9. 'Residential Management', op. cit., p.60.
10. 'The Problem of Homeless Children', op. cit.
11. Ibid.
12. Ibid.

13. Ibid.
14. 'On Influencing and Being Influenced' (1941), Winnicott 1964a, p.204.
15. 'The Problem of Homeless Children', op. cit.
16. Ibid.
17. Ibid.
18. Introduction, Winnicott 1965, p.10.
19. 'Home Again' (1945), Winnicott 1984, p.51.
20. Idem.
21. Ibid., p.52.
22. 'Discussion of War Aims' (1940), Winnicott 1987a, pp.210–20.
23. Ibid., p.216.
24. 'Some Thoughts on the Meaning of the Word Democracy' (1950), Winnicott 1964b, pp.155–69.
25. 'Discussion of War Aims', op. cit., p.214.
26. 'The Capacity to be Alone' (1958), Winnicott 1965, pp.34–5. See 'Ego-Orgasm in Bisexual Love' (1974), Khan 1979, for further commentary on this notion that Winnicott never developed.
27. 'Appetite and Emotional Disorder' (1936), Winnicott 1958, pp.33–51. This quotation p.49.
28. 'The Observation of Infants in a Set Situation' (1941), Winnicott 1958, pp.52–69.
29. 'Appetite and Emotional Disorder', op. cit., pp.45–6.
30. Ibid., p.47.
31. 'The Observation of Infants', op. cit., p.67.
32. Idem.
33. Idem.
34. 'Primitive Emotional Development' (1945), Winnicott 1958, pp.145–56.
35. 'Notes on Some Schizoid Mechanisms' (1946), in *Envy and Gratitude* by Melanie Klein (London: The Hogarth Press and The Institute of Psycho-Analysis, 1975).
36. 'Primitive Emotional Development', op. cit., p.145. (In Winnicott 1988, p.2, Winnicott describes himself as being 'gradually lured into the treatment of the more psychotic type of adult patient'.)
37. Ibid., p.147.
38. Ibid., p.148.
39. Idem.
40. Ibid., p.149.
41. Winnicott refers to this elsewhere, using a term from Heidegger, as 'what might be called "in-dwelling": the achievement of a close and easy relationship between the psyche and the body, and body functioning', Winnicott 1965, p.68.
42. 'The Mind and its Relation to the Psyche-Soma' (1949), Winnicott 1958, p.244.

43. 'The First Year of Life' (1958), Winnicott 1964b, p.6.
44. Idem.
45. 'Primitive Emotional Development', op. cit., p. 149.
46. 'The First Year of Life', op. cit., p.6.
47. 'Primitive Emotional Development', op. cit., p.151.
48. 'Ego Integration in Child Development' (1962), Winnicott 1965, p.61.
49. 'Primitive Emotional Development', op. cit., p.150.
50. Ibid., p.151.
51. Idem.
52. Idem.
53. 'Group Influences and the Maladjusted Child' (1955), Winnicott 1964b, p.148.
54. Ibid., p.154.
55. Ibid., p.152.
56. Ibid., p.153.
57. Idem.
58. Idem.
59. Quoted in Davis and Wallbridge 1983, pp.67–8.
60. Idem.
61. 'Paediatrics and Psychiatry' (1948), Winnicott 1958, p.159.
62. 'Primitive Emotional Development', op. cit., p.154.
63. Idem.
64. 'Hate in the Countertransference' (1947), Winnicott 1958, pp.194–203.
65. Ibid., p.198.
66. Idem.
67. Ibid., p.199.
68. Ibid., p.200.
69. Ibid., p.203.
70. 'Reparation in Respect of Mother's Organized Defence against Depression' (1948), Winnicott 1958, pp.91–6.
71. Ibid., p.96.
72. Ibid., p.93.
73. Ibid., p.95.
74. Ibid., p.92.
75. Ibid., p.93.
76. 'The Mind and its Relation to the Psyche-Soma', op. cit.
77. Ibid., p.245.
78. 'Birth Memories, Birth Trauma, and Anxiety' (1949), Winnicott 1958, pp.183–4.
79. Idem.
80. Idem.
81. 'The Mind and its Relation to the Psyche-Soma', op. cit., p.246.
82. 'The First Year of Life', op. cit., p.7.

83. 'The Mind', op. cit., p.248.
84. Ibid., p.254. In Winnicott 1988, Winnicott writes that 'Human nature is not a matter of mind and body – it is a matter of inter-related psyche and soma, with the mind as a flourish on the edge of psychosomatic functioning' (p.26). But to complicate the issue he also suggests that there is 'an organization of this relationship [between psyche and soma] coming from that which we call the mind' (p.11), which either confers an omnipotently managerial function upon the mind, or implies that the mind organizes the psyche-soma in the service of representation. Lack of conventional conceptual clarity always points to an essential perplexity in his work.
85. Little 1985.

4. *The Appearing Self*

1. 'Advising Parents' (1957), Winnicott 1964b, p.119.
2. 'The Contribution of Psycho-Analysis to Midwifery' (1957), Winnicott 1964b, p.107.
3. 'The Family Affected by Depressive Illness in One or Both Parents' (1958), Winnicott 1964b, p.55.
4. 'Theoretical Statement of the Field of Child Psychiatry' (1958), Winnicott 1964b, p.98.
5. Rycroft 1985, p.114.
6. In *Envy and Gratitude* by Melanie Klein (London: The Hogarth Press and The Institute of Psycho-Analysis, 1975), pp.176–235.
7. 'A Study of Envy and Gratitude', Comment by D. W. Winnicott, privately circulated, 24 February 1956.
8. Ibid.
9. 'Psychoanalytic Studies of the Personality', *International Journal of Psycho-Analysis*, 34: 1953.
10. Ibid.
11. 'Primary Maternal Preoccupation' (1956), Winnicott 1958, pp.300–5.
12. 'The Anti-Social Tendency' (1956), ibid., pp.306–15.
13. 'Transitional Objects and Transitional Phenomena' (1951), ibid., pp.229–42.
14. 'Aggression in Relation to Emotional Development' (1950), ibid., pp.204–18.
15. *British Medical Journal*, 12 June 1954, p.1363.
16. In 'A Personal View of the Kleinian Contribution' (1962), Winnicott 1965, Winnicott writes that he 'simply cannot find value in [Freud's] idea of a Death Instinct' (p.177), and lists under Klein's 'more doubtful contributions' her 'retaining a use of the theory of the Life and Death Instincts' (p.178).
17. See note 14 above.

18. 'The Depressive Position and Normal Development' (1954), Winnicott 1958, pp.262–77.
19. 'Psychoanalysis and the Sense of Guilt' (1957), Winnicott 1965, pp.15–28.
20. 'The First Year of Life' (1958), Winnicott 1964b, p.12.
21. Idem.
22. 'Classification' (1959–64), Winnicott 1965, p.127.
23. *Standard Edition*, XXI, p.122.
24. 'Aggression', op. cit., p.210.
25. Ibid., p.206.
26. 'The Depressive Position', op. cit., p.263.
27. 'Psychoanalysis and the Sense of Guilt', op. cit., p.24.
28. Idem.
29. Ibid., p.23.
30. 'The Depressive Position', op. cit., p.268.
31. 'Aggression', op. cit., p.214.
32. Idem.
33. Ibid., p.215.
34. Idem.
35. Idem.
36. Ibid., p.216.
37. Ibid., p.217.
38. Idem.
39. 'The Depressive Position', op. cit., p.268.
40. For examples of Kleinian views on aesthetics see Hanna Segal, *The Work of Hanna Segal: a Kleinian Approach to Clinical Practice* (New York and London: Aronson, 1981), chapters 16–18; Adrian Stokes, *The Critical Writings of Adrian Stokes*, volume 3 (London: Thames and Hudson, 1978); Donald Meltzer, *Sexual States of Mind* (Perthshire: Clunie Press, 1973), chapter 24; R. E. Money-Kyrle, *Man's Picture of His World: A Psycho-Analytic Study* (London: Duckworth, 1961), chapter 7.
41. 'Reparation in Respect of Mother's Organized Defence against Depression' (1948), Winnicott 1958, p.91.
42. 'The Depressive Position', op. cit., p.270.
43. 'Psychoanalysis', op. cit., p.26. A more elaborate account of some of the ideas can be found in Phillips 1988.
44. 'Aggression', op. cit., p.208.
45. 'Transitional Objects', op. cit.
46. Ibid., p.231.
47. Ibid., p.233.
48. 'The Deprived Child and how he can be Compensated for Loss of Family Life' (1950), Winnicott 1964b, pp.143–4.
49. 'Transitional Objects', op. cit., p.230.

50. Idem.
51. Ibid., p.231.
52. Idem.
53. 'The Deprived Child', op. cit., p.135.
54. See notes 12 and 11 respectively.
55. 'Transitional Objects', p.240.
56. Ibid., p.239.
57. In 'Living Creatively' (1970), Winnicott 1987a, p.47, Winnicott writes: 'If one has been happy, one can bear distress. It is the same when we say that a baby cannot be weaned unless he or she has had the breast, or breast equivalent. There is no disillusionment (acceptance of the Reality Principle) except on a basis of illusion.'
58. 'Transitional Objects', p.240.
59. 'Primary Maternal Preoccupation', p.303.
60. Ibid., p.304.
61. Idem.
62. Ibid., p.303.
63. Ibid., p.304.
64. Ibid., pp.304–5.
65. Idem.
66. 'The Mother's Contribution to Society' (Postscript to Winnicott 1957), Winnicott 1987a, p.123.

5. Real-making

1. 'The Location of Cultural Experience' (1967), Winnicott 1971a, p.116.
2. 'Ego Distortion in Terms of True and False Self' (1960), Winnicott 1965, p.148.
3. 'Mirror-Role of Mother and Family in Child Development' (1967), Winnicott 1971a, pp.137–8.
4. 'The Relationship of a Mother to her Baby at the Beginning' (1960), Winnicott 1964b, pp.17–18.
5. 'Mirror-Role', op. cit., pp.130–8.
6. 'The Use of an Object and Relating through Identifications' (1969), Winnicott 1971a, pp.101–11.
7. 'Ego Distortion', op. cit., pp.140–52.
8. Écrits: a Selection, translated by Alan Sheridan (London: Tavistock, 1977), pp.1–7.
9. 'Mirror-Role', op. cit., p.134.
10. 'The Use of an Object', op. cit., p.106.
11. Idem.
12. 'Ego Distortion', op. cit., p.152. For a sceptical view of Winnicott's notions of creativity see Pontalis's remarks in Clancier and Kalmanovitch 1987: 'Trying to get everybody to believe that there is a

treasure inside him is a false scent. To say, as Winnicott does, even with humour, that one can be as creative in frying eggs as Schumann composing a sonata, don't you find that rather excessive?' (p.143.)

13. 'The Concept of a Healthy Individual' (1967), Winnicott 1987a, p.23.
14. All further quotations in this chapter are from 'Ego Distortion', op. cit.
15. 'Ego Distortion', p.145.
16. Ibid., p.150.
17. Idem.

6. The Play of Interpretation

1. 'The Theory of the Parent–Infant Relationship' (1960), Winnicott 1965, p.40.
2. 'Child Analysis in the Latency Period' (1958), Winnicott 1965, p.117.
3. Ibid., p.122.
4. *Standard Edition*, XII, p.139.
5. 'Providing for the Child in Health and in Crisis' (1962), Winnicott 1965, p.68.
6. 'The Aims of Psycho-Analytical Treatment' (1962), Winnicott 1965, p.167.
7. 'The Theory', op. cit., p.50.
8. Idem.
9. 'Ego Integration in Child Development' (1962), Winnicott 1965, pp.59–60.
10. 'The Aims of Psycho-Analytical Treatment' (1962), Winnicott 1965, p.167.
11. Idem.
12. 'Playing: a Theoretical Statement' (1971), Winnicott 1971a, p.59.
13. Introduction, Winnicott 1971b, pp.9–10.
14. 'Morals and Education' (1963), Winnicott 1965, p.100.
15. 'Playing: a Theoretical Statement', op. cit., p.48.
16. 'Communicating and Not Communicating Leading to a Study of Certain Opposites' (1963), Winnicott 1965, pp.179–92.
17. Ibid., p.187.
18. Ibid., p.190.
19. 'Morals and Education', op. cit., p.105.
20. 'Communicating and Not Communicating', op. cit., p.189.
21. Ibid., p.187.
22. Ibid., p.179.
23. 'The Capacity to be Alone' (1958), Winnicott 1965, pp.29–36.
24. 'Communicating and Not Communicating', op. cit., p.188.
25. Ibid., p.192.
26. Idem.

27. Ibid., pp.189–90.
28. Ibid., p.187.
29. Ibid., p.183.
30. Ibid., p.184. This may be one way of understanding the pleasure of ordinary, as opposed to compulsive, masturbation. The idea of developing a capacity for satisfying masturbatory experience has never, for some reason, found a place in psychoanalytic theory.
31. Idem.
32. Idem.
33. Ibid., p.187.
34. 'On Influencing and Being Influenced' (1941), Winnicott 1964a, pp.199–204.
35. 'Communicating and Not Communicating', op. cit., p.187.
36. Ibid., p.185.
37. But in this paper Winnicott implicitly contrasts the adult artist with the developing child. While for the artist there is 'the still more urgent need not to be found', Winnicott offers us 'a picture of a child establishing a private self that is not communicating, and at the same time wanting to communicate and to be found. It is a sophisticated game of hide-and-seek in which it is joy to be hidden but disaster not to be found' (p.185). It is as though there is a growing developmental need to conceive of a space inside the Self that cannot be filled, or entered into, by another person (or oneself as another person), and that must be recognized as such.
38. *International Journal of Psycho-Analysis*, 45: 1964.

BIBLIOGRAPHY

Winnicott: Principal Works

Winnicott 1931: *Clinical Notes on Disorders of Childhood.* London: Heinemann.

Winnicott 1957a: *The Child and the Family: First Relationships.* London: Tavistock.

Winnicott 1957b: *The Child and the Outside World: Studies in Developing Relationships.* London: Tavistock.

Winnicott 1958: *Collected Papers: Through Paediatrics to Psycho-Analysis.* London: Tavistock; New York: Basic Books.

Winnicott 1964a: *The Child, the Family, and the Outside World.* Harmondsworth: Penguin Books.

Winnicott 1964b: *The Family and Individual Development.* London: Tavistock.

Winnicott 1965: *The Maturational Processes and the Facilitating Environment: Studies in the Theory of Emotional Development.* London: The Hogarth Press and The Institute of Psycho-Analysis.

Winnicott 1971a: *Playing and Reality.* London: Tavistock.

Winnicott 1971b: *Therapeutic Consultations in Child Psychiatry.* London: The Hogarth Press and The Institute of Psycho-Analysis.

Winnicott 1977: *The Piggle: an Account of the Psychoanalytic Treatment of a Little Girl.* London: The Hogarth Press and The Institute of Psycho-Analysis.

Winnicott 1984: *Deprivation and Delinquency.* London: Tavistock.

Winnicott 1986: *Holding and Interpretation: Fragment of*

an Analysis. London: The Hogarth Press and The Institute of Psycho-Analysis.

Winnicott 1987a: *Home is Where We Start From: Essays by a Psychoanalyst*. London: Pelican Books.

Winnicott 1987b: *The Spontaneous Gesture: Selected Letters of D. W. Winnicott*, edited by F. Robert Rodman. Cambridge, Massachusetts, and London: Harvard University Press.

Winnicott 1988: *Human Nature*. London: Free Association Books.

Books on Winnicott

S. Grolnick *et al.* (eds.), *Between Reality and Fantasy*. London and New York: Jason Aronson, 1978.

M. Davis and D. Wallbridge, *Boundary and Space: an introduction to the Work of D. W. Winnicott*. Harmondsworth: Penguin Books, 1983.

A. Clancier and J. Kalmanovitch, *Winnicott and Paradox: from Birth to Creation*. London: Tavistock, 1987.

Books and Articles relating to Winnicott

This section includes texts that use Winnicott's writings in an illuminating way.

Roland Barthes, *A Lover's Discourse: Fragments*, trans. Richard Howard. London: Jonathan Cape, 1979.

Christopher Bollas, *The Shadow of the Object: Psychoanalysis of the Unthought Known*. London: Free Association Books, 1987.

Michael Eigen, 'The Area of Faith in Winnicott, Lacan, and

Bion', *International Journal of Psycho-Analysis*, 62, pp.413–33 (1981).

— 'Guntrip's Analysis with Winnicott', *Contemporary Psychoanalysis*, 17, pp.103–17 (1981).

— *The Psychotic Core*. London and New Jersey: Jason Aronson, 1986.

R. Gaddini, 'Bion's Catastrophic Change and Winnicott's Breakdown', *Revista di Psicoanalisi*, pp.3–4, Rome, (1981).

André Green, *On Private Madness*. London: The Hogarth Press and the Institute of Psycho-Analysis, 1986.

J. Greenberg and S. Mitchell, *Object Relations in Psychoanalytic Theory*. Cambridge, Massachusetts, and London: Harvard University Press, 1983.

Ralph R. Greenson, *Explorations in Psychoanalysis*. New York: International Universities Press, 1978.

Phyllis Grosskurth, *Melanie Klein: Her World and Her Work*. London: Hodder and Stoughton, 1987.

H. Guntrip, 'My Experience of Analysis with Fairbairn and Winnicott', *International Review of Psycho-Analysis*, 2, pp.145–56 (1975).

Geoffrey H. Hartman, *Criticism in the Wilderness: the Study of Literature Today*. New Haven: Yale University Press, 1980.

L. D. Jacobson, *Development of and in the Group* (unpublished PhD dissertation: The City University of New York, 1985).

M. Masud R. Khan, *The Privacy of the Self*. London: The Hogarth Press and The Institute of Psycho-Analysis, 1974.

— Introduction to D. W. Winnicott, *Through Paediatrics to Psycho-Analysis*. London: The Hogarth Press and The Institute of Psycho-Analysis, 1975.

— *Alienation in Perversions*. London: The Hogarth Press and The Institute of Psycho-Analysis, 1979.

— *Hidden Selves.* London: The Hogarth Press and The Institute of Psycho-Analysis, 1983.

— Introduction to D. W. Winnicott, *Holding and Interpretation: Fragment of an Analysis.* London: The Hogarth Press and The Institute of Psycho-Analysis, 1986.

Gregorio Kohon (ed.), *The British School of Psychoanalysis: the Independent Tradition.* London: Free Association Books, 1986.

Margaret Little, *Transference Neurosis and Transference Psychosis.* London and New York: Jason Aronson, 1981.

— 'Winnicott Working in Areas Where Psychotic Anxieties Predominate: a Personal Record', *Free Associations*, no. 3 (1985).

Peter Lomas, *True and False Experience.* London: Allen Lane, 1973.

— *The Case for a Personal Psychotherapy.* Oxford: Oxford University Press, 1981.

— *The Limits of Interpretation: What's Wrong with Psychoanalysis?* Harmondsworth: Penguin Books, 1987.

Maud Mannoni, *D'un impossible à l'autre.* Paris: Seuil, 1982.

Perry Meisel and Walter Kendrick (eds.), *Bloomsbury/Freud: the Letters of James and Alix Strachey 1924–1925.* London: Chatto and Windus, 1986.

Marion Milner, *The Hands of the Living God: an Account of a Psycho-Analytic Treatment.* London: The Hogarth Press and The Institute of Psycho-Analysis, 1969.

— *The Suppressed Madness of Sane Men: Forty-four Years of Exploring Psychoanalysis.* London: Tavistock Publications in association with The Institute of Psycho-Analysis, 1987.

Thomas H. Ogden, *The Matrix of the Mind: Object Relations and the Psychoanalytic Dialogue.* London and New Jersey: Jason Aronson, 1986.

Adam Phillips, ' "That Dreadful Universal Thing": a Review

Article', *Journal of Child Psychotherapy*, vol. II, no. 1 (1985).

— 'On Composure', *Raritan*, vol. V, no. 4 (1986).

— 'On Being Bored', *Raritan*, vol. VI, no.2 (1986).

— 'Le Risque de la solitude', *Nouvelle Revue de Psychoanalyse* (Autumn 1987).

— 'On Moral Surprises: a Winnicottian Approach to Moral Development', *Raritan*, vol. VIII, no. 1 (1988).

Richard Poirier, 'Frost, Winnicott, Burke', *Raritan*, vol. 2, no.2 (1982).

J.-B. Pontalis, *Frontiers in Psychoanalysis: Between the Dream and Psychic Pain*. London: The Hogarth Press and The Institute of Psycho-Analysis, 1981.

Barry Richards (ed.), *Capitalism and Infancy: Essays on Psychoanalysis and Politics*. London: Free Association Books, 1984.

Charles Rycroft, *Psychoanalysis and Beyond*. London: Chatto and Windus, 1985.

Murray M. Schwartz, 'Critic, Define Thyself', in *Psychoanalysis and the Question of the Text*, ed. Geoffrey H. Hartman. Baltimore and London: Johns Hopkins University Press, 1978.

Harold F. Searles, *Countertransference and Related Subjects: Selected Papers*. New York: International Universities Press, 1979.

Daniel N. Stern, *The Interpersonal World of the Infant: a View from Psychoanalysis and Developmental Psychology*. New York: Basic Books, 1985.

Neville Symington, *The Analytic Experience: Lectures from the Tavistock*. London: Free Association Books, 1986.

Frances Tustin, *Autistic States in Children*. London and Boston: Routledge and Kegan Paul, 1981.

— *Autistic Barriers in Neurotic Patients*. London: Karnac Books, 1986.

INDEX

(Since references to mothers and infants can be found on virtually every page they are not indexed.)

Index

Index

Index